T0195200

Office-Based Procedures: Part II

Editors

KARL T. CLEBAK
ALEXIS REEDY-COOPER

PRIMARY CARE:
CLINICS IN OFFICE PRACTICE

www.primarycare.theclinics.com

Consulting Editor
JOEL J. HEIDELBAUGH

March 2022 • Volume 49 • Number 1

ELSEVIER

1600 John F. Kennedy Boulevard • Suite 1800 • Philadelphia, Pennsylvania, 19103-2899

http://www.theclinics.com

PRIMARY CARE: CLINICS IN OFFICE PRACTICE Volume 49, Number 1
March 2022 ISSN 0095-4543, ISBN-13: 978-0-323-80919-1

Editor: Katerina Heidhausen
Developmental Editor: Jessica Cañaberal

Primary Care: Clinics in Office Practice (ISSN: 0095-4543) is published quarterly by Elsevier Inc., 360 Park Avenue South, New York, NY 10010-1710. Months of issue are March, June, September, and December. Periodicals postage paid at New York, NY and additional mailing offices. Subscription prices are $260.00 per year (US individuals), $672.00 (US institutions), $100.00 (US students), $312.00 (Canadian individuals), $696.00 (Canadian institutions), $100.00 (Canadian students), $368.00 (international individuals), $696.00 (international institutions), and $175.00 (international students). Foreign air speed delivery is included in all *Clinics* subscription prices. All prices are subject to change without notice. POSTMASTER: Send address changes to *Primary Care: Clinics in Office Practice*, Elsevier Periodicals Customer Service, 11830 Westline Industrial Drive, St. Louis, MO 63146. Customer Service Health Sciences Division, Subscription Customer Service, 3251 Riverport Lane, Maryland Heights, MO 63043. **Customer Service: 1-800-654-2452 (U.S. and Canada); 314-447-8871 (outside U.S. and Canada). Fax: 314-447-8029. E-mail: journalscustomerservice-usa@elsevier.com (for print support); journalsonlinesupport-usa@elsevier.com (for online support).**

Reprints. For copies of 100 or more, of articles in this publication, please contact the Commercial Reprints Department, Elsevier Inc., 360 Park Avenue South, New York, NY 10010-1710. Tel. 212-633-3874; Fax: 212-633-3820; E-mail: reprints@elsevier.com.

Primary Care: Clinics in Office Practice is covered in *MEDLINE/PubMed (Index Medicus)* and *EMBASE/Excerpta Medica, Current Contents/Clinical Medicine,* and *ISI/BIOMED.*

Contributors

CONSULTING EDITOR

JOEL J. HEIDELBAUGH, MD, FAAFP, FACG
Clinical Professor, Departments of Family Medicine and Urology, Director of Medical Student Education and Clerkship, Director, Department of Family Medicine, University of Michigan Medical School, Ann Arbor, Michigan; Ypsilanti Health Center, Ypsilanti, Michigan

EDITORS

KARL T. CLEBAK, MD, MHA, FAAFP
Associate Professor, Program Director, Family and Community Medicine Residency Program, Department of Family and Community Medicine, Penn State Health Milton S. Hershey Medical Center, Hershey, Pennsylvania; Penn State College of Medicine, Harrisburg, Pennsylvania

ALEXIS REEDY-COOPER, MD, MPH
Associate Professor, Program Director, Family and Community Medicine Residency Program, Department of Family and Community Medicine, Penn State Health St. Joseph Medical Center, Reading, Pennsylvania

AUTHORS

JUSTIN BAILEY, MD, FAAFP
Procedural Institute Director, Family Medicine Residency of Idaho, Boise, Idaho; Associate Professor, Department of Family Medicine, University of Washington School of Medicine

KEVIN BERNSTEIN, MD, MMS, CAQSM
Assistant Professor, Department of Orthopedics and Sports Medicine, United States Naval Academy, Annapolis, Maryland

CHRISTOPHER L. BOSWELL, MD
Assistant Professor, Department of Family Medicine, Mayo Clinic, Rochester, Minnesota

JAIME K. BOWMAN, MD, FAAFP
Clinical Associate Professor, Department of Medical Education and Clinical Sciences, Washington State University, Spokane, Washington

PETER CASHIO, MD, MS
Founder, Code 1 Concierge Care, Austin, Texas; Baptist Emergency Hospital, Schertz, Texas

ERIN CATHCART, MD
Assistant Professor, Department of Family Medicine and Community Health, University of Massachusetts Medical School, North Worcester, Massachusetts

KARL T. CLEBAK, MD, MHA, FAAFP
Associate Professor, Program Director, Family and Community Medicine Residency Program, Department of Family and Community Medicine, Penn State Health Milton S. Hershey Medical Center, Hershey, Pennsylvania; Penn State College of Medicine, Harrisburg, Pennsylvania

JASON CROAD, DO
Assistant Professor, Associate Program Director, Department of Family and Community Medicine Residency Program, Penn State College of Medicine, Hershey, Pennsylvania

JARED DUBEY, DO
Assistant Professor, Department of Family Medicine and Community Health, University of Wisconsin-Madison School of Medicine and Public Health, Madison, Wisconsin

NATHAN FALK, MD, MBA
Associate Professor, Family Medicine Residency Director, Florida State University, Winter Haven, Florida

MICHAEL FITZGERALD, DO
Department of Family and Community Medicine, University of Kentucky, Lexington, Kentucky

BRADY FLESHMAN, MD
Assistant Professor, Department of Orthopedic Surgery and Sports Medicine, University of Missouri, Columbia, Missouri

AMRIT GREENE, MD
Assistant Professor of Dermatology, Penn State Hershey Medical Center, Hershey, Pennsylvania

JASON D. GREENWOOD, MD, MS
Instructor, Department of Family Medicine, Mayo Clinic, Rochester, Minnesota

SMRITI GUPTA, MD
Family Medicine Resident, Department of Family and Community Medicine, Penn State Health, State College, Pennsylvania

LEESHA A. HELM, MD, MPH
Assistant Professor of Family and Community Medicine, Penn State Hershey Medical Center, Hershey, Pennsylvania

MATTHEW F. HELM, MD
Assistant Professor of Dermatology, Penn State Hershey Medical Center, Hershey, Pennsylvania

HANNAH HORNSBY, MD
Family Medicine Resident Physician, Department of Family Medicine, Offutt AFB/UNMC Family Medicine Residency Program, University of Nebraska Medical Center College of Medicine, Nebraska Medical Center, Omaha, Nebraska

KIMBERLY KAISER, MD
Associate Professor, Department of Orthopaedic Surgery and Sports Medicine, University of Kentucky, Lexington, Kentucky

ASHLEY KOONTZ, DO
Family Medicine Resident, Department of Family and Community Medicine, Penn State Health, Hershey, Pennsylvania

LINDSAY LAFFERTY, MD
Assistant Professor, Departments of Family and Community Medicine, and Orthopedics and Rehabilitation, Penn State Health, Hershey, Pennsylvania

GEORGE LE, MD
Sports Medicine Fellow, Harbor-UCLA Medical Center, Torrance, California

CHARLES MADDEN, MD
Staff Physician, Spectrum Health Big Rapids Hospital Family Medicine, Big Rapids, Michigan

T. JASON MEREDITH, MD
Sports Medicine Fellowship Director, Assistant Professor and Associate Program Director, Department of Family Medicine, UNMC Family Medicine Residency Program, University of Nebraska Medical Center College of Medicine, Nebraska Medical Center, Omaha, Nebraska

STEPHEN P. MERRY, MD, MPH
Assistant Professor, Department of Family Medicine, Mayo Clinic, Rochester, Minnesota

JOHN MESSMER, MD
Professor, Department of Family and Community Medicine, Penn State College of Medicine, Hershey, Pennsylvania

ASHLEY MORRISON, MD
Assistant Professor, Department of Family and Community Medicine, Penn State College of Medicine, Hershey, Pennsylvania

AMY MOYERS, MD
Assistant Professor, Department of Family Medicine, WVU Medicine, Morgantown, West Virginia

ROLAND NEWMAN II, DO
Assistant Professor, Associate Program Director, Department of Family and Community Medicine Residency Program, Penn State College of Medicine, Harrisburg, Pennsylvania

CAYCE ONKS, DO, MS, ATC
Associate Professor, Departments of Family and Community Medicine, and Orthopedics and Rehabilitation, Penn State Health, Hershey, Pennsylvania

MICHAEL PARTIN, MD
Assistant Professor of Family and Community Medicine, Penn State Hershey Medical Center, Hershey, Pennsylvania

BERNADETTE PENDERGRAPH, MD
Sports Medicine Fellowship Director, Harbor-UCLA Medical Center, Torrance, California

PRABHAT K. POKHREL, MS, MD, PhD, FAAFP
Program Director, Family Medicine Residency, Chair, Department of Family Medicine, McLaren Flint, Flint, Michigan

KATHLEEN ROBERTS, MD
Assistant Professor, Department of Family and Community Medicine, University of Kentucky, Lexington, Kentucky

BRIAN SHIAN, MD
Department of Family Medicine, Clinical Associate Professor, University of Iowa Carver College of Medicine, Iowa City, Iowa

BENJAMIN SILVERBERG, MD, MSc
Associate Professor, Department of Emergency Medicine, Associate Professor, Department of Family Medicine, WVU Medicine, Medical Director, Division of Physician Assistant Studies, Department of Human Performance, West Virginia University School of Medicine, Morgantown, West Virginia

BENJAMIN I. WAINBLAT, MD
Chief Resident, Department of Family and Community Health, Marshall University Joan C. Edwards School of Medicine, Huntington, West Virginia

KEVIN WILE, MD
Assistant Professor, Department of Family and Community Medicine Residency Program, Penn State College of Medicine, Middletown, Pennsylvania

Contents

Foreword: You're a Dermatologist Too? xi

Joel J. Heidelbaugh

Preface: Procedures in Primary Care: Meeting the Comprehensive Needs of Our Patients Where They Are xiii

Karl T. Clebak and Alexis Reedy-Cooper

Skin Biopsy Techniques 1

Jason D. Greenwood, Stephen P. Merry, and Christopher L. Boswell

Because many skin lesions and disorders can appear similar, primary care clinicians often struggle to diagnose them definitively without histopathologic information obtained from a biopsy. This review article explains how to decide whether a lesion should be biopsied and what type of biopsy technique to use and then outlines the stepwise approach to each of the most common skin biopsy techniques: shave, saucerization, punch, fusiform, and subcutaneous nodule biopsies. Finally, potential pitfalls and complications are discussed so the clinician can avoid those and can provide a cosmetically acceptable result from these common outpatient procedures.

A Stitch in Time: Operative and Nonoperative Laceration Repair Techniques 23

Benjamin Silverberg, Amy Moyers, Benjamin I. Wainblat, Peter Cashio, and Kevin Bernstein

Before repairing a laceration, consider the mechanism and severity of the injury. Gentle irrigation of the wound helps to remove microscopic infectious agents and larger debris. Not all foreign bodies are visible in plain radiographs. Certain wounds may be allowed to heal without operative intervention, but most patients prefer an approach using suture thread or tissue adhesive. Prophylaxis against tetanus, rabies, and/or bacterial infection should be considered. Clinical assessment of each wound is important to guide decisions about technique, anesthetic, suture material, and the interval period before nonabsorbable equipment can be removed.

Abscess Incision and Drainage 39

Jaime K. Bowman

An abscess is a localized collection of purulent material surrounded by inflammation and granulation in response to an infectious source. Most simple abscesses can be diagnosed upon clinical examination and safely be managed in the ambulatory office with incision and drainage. Wound culture and antibiotics do not improve healing, but packing wounds larger than 5 cm may reduce recurrence and complications.

Assorted Skin Procedures: Foreign Body Removal, Cryotherapy, Electrosurgery, and Treatment of Keloids   47

Roland Newman II, Karl T. Clebak, Jason Croad, Kevin Wile, and Erin Cathcart

Clinicians in the primary care setting will encounter various different skin conditions requiring procedural intervention. There are many different procedural approaches to treatment. Knowing which modalities are available and best suited to handle a particular skin lesion allows for flexibility for patient and clinician. Although some treatment modalities may be used more than others, it is helpful to be at least familiar with basic in office skin procedures such as removal of foreign bodies, cryotherapy, electrosurgery, and treatment of keloids, as these procedures are helpful in addressing the wide variety of the most commonly encountered skin issues in primary care.

Nail and Foot Procedures   63

Justin Bailey

Primary care physicians provide a wide variety of treatments and conditions affecting the foot. This article discusses the removal of toenails, both full and partial removal. Subungual hematoma/Subungual blistering evacuation as well as wart, corn, callus, and blister management will also be discussed.

Management of Chronic Wounds   85

Ashley Morrison, Charles Madden, and John Messmer

 Video content accompanies this article at http://www.primarycare. theclinics.com.

Chronic wounds originate from venous hypertension, arterial insufficiency, or pressure-induced ischemia. Determination of the type and associated causes and contributory conditions is essential for the diagnosis and management of these common conditions.

Dermoscopy in Primary Care   99

Prabhat K. Pokhrel, Matthew F. Helm, Amrit Greene, Leesha A. Helm, and Michael Partin

Dermoscopy is a noninvasive technique that allows in vivo magnification of the skin structures and helps in visualizing microscopic features that are imperceptible to the naked eye. Dermoscopy is not a substitute for biopsy and histopathologic evaluation, but is an important tool that can help increase diagnostic sensitivity and specificity of cutaneous lesions. Dermoscopy increases the diagnostic sensitivity compared with naked eye examination. A significant improvement in diagnostic accuracy for benign and malignant lesions has been reported among family medicine physicians after an introductory training course on dermoscopy.

Large and Intermediate Joint Injections: Olecranon Bursa, Greater Trochanteric Bursa, Medial and Lateral Epicondyle Peritendinous Injections   119

Kimberly Kaiser, Michael Fitzgerald, Brady Fleshman, and Kathleen Roberts

Olecranon bursitis, greater trochanteric bursitis, medial epicondylosis, and lateral epicondylosis are common diagnoses encountered in primary care and sports medicine clinics. This section explores the anatomy, clinical presentation, evaluation, procedural techniques, and management to effectively treat these common conditions.

Small Joint, Tendon, and Myofascial Injections   131

Lindsay Lafferty, Smriti Gupta, Ashley Koontz, and Cayce Onks

Small joint, peritendinous, and myofascial injections can be used for both diagnostic and therapeutic purposes. This article reviews injections for carpal tunnel, first dorsal compartment, trigger finger, ganglion cysts, trigger point, and plantar fascia. Necessary equipment should be gathered before the procedure and informed consent should be obtained. Indications, contraindications, and possible complications should be reviewed. Complete understanding of anatomy before injection is paramount. The injection technique should minimize risk of infection. There are no evidence-based postinjection protocols, and outcomes vary depending on the site and medication injected.

Managing Fractures and Sprains   145

Nathan Falk, Bernadette Pendergraph, T. Jason Meredith, George Le, and Hannah Hornsby

 Video content accompanies this article at http://www.primarycare. theclinics.com.

Primary care physicians are often the first to evaluate patients with extremity injuries. Identification of fractures and sprains and their proper management is paramount. After appropriate imaging is obtained, immobilization and determination of definitive management, either nonoperative or operative, is critical. Appropriate immobilization is imperative to injury healing. Nonsurgical management of upper extremity fractures often uses slings, short-term splinting, gutter splints, and/or short or long arm casts. Initial fracture stabilization of the lower extremity is usually accomplished with a posterior splint. Definitive management usually uses controlled ankle movement walker boots, hard-sole shoes, or casting.

Point-of-Care Ultrasound for Musculoskeletal Injection and Clinical Evaluation   163

Jared Dubey and Brian Shian

 Video content accompanies this article at http://www.primarycare. theclinics.com.

Primary care is poised to become the latest field to widely adopt Point-of-Care Ultrasound (POCUS). POCUS offers many benefits for efficient diagnosis and treatment of common conditions encountered in the clinical setting. This article reviews POCUS basics and presents evidence and best practices for the use of POCUS for musculoskeletal-guided injection and clinical evaluation of the heart, lungs, abdominal aorta, lower extremity deep veins, soft tissue infection, and foreign bodies.

PRIMARY CARE:
CLINICS IN OFFICE PRACTICE

FORTHCOMING ISSUES

June 2022
Diabetes Management
Lenard Salzberg, *Editor*

September 2022
Chronic Pain Management
David O' Gurek, *Editor*

December 2022
Telehealth
Joel Heidelbaugh, Kathryn M. Harmes, and Robert J. Heizelman, *Editors*

RECENT ISSUES

December 2021
Office-Based Procedures: Part I
J. Lane Wilson and Jonathon Firnhaber, *Editors*

September 2021
Common Pediatric Issues in Primary Care
Luz M. Fernandez and Jonathan A. Becker, *Editors*

June 2021
LGBTQ+ Health
Jessica Lapinski and Kristine M. Diaz, *Editors*

SERIES OF RELATED INTEREST

Medical Clinics (http://www.medical.theclinics.com)
Physician Assistant Clinics (https://www.physicianassistant.theclinics.com)

Foreword

You're a Dermatologist Too?

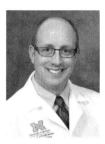

Joel J. Heidelbaugh, MD, FAAFP, FACG
Consulting Editor

Since I completed my residency training in 1999, I have enjoyed a challenging and rewarding career in academic family medicine. While my original plan was to go to medical school and become a surgeon, like many medical students in their clerkship year I found myself liking essentially everything and struggling to commit to a single subspecialty for fear that I would be narrowing my focus in patient care. I realized during my residency that family medicine gave me the opportunity to develop a broad expertise in all areas of medicine and to become skilled in many procedures. Office-based procedures greatly add to the diversity of what clinicians can offer within their practices and can improve practice margins through additional revenue that would be diverted to subspecialty care. Procedures can also help to define a niche within one's practice, and our patient satisfaction surveys have shown that patients greatly appreciate when their family physician can provide a service—with the same level of skill, expertise, and outcomes as a subspecialist–within the primary care practice without having to wait for a referral.

In addition to developing skills in performing procedures in these areas, enhancing our knowledge of the conditions that benefit from procedural intervention also augments our knowledge of relevant differential diagnoses and therapeutic options. For example, I have always performed many dermatologic procedures in my practice, and as I have a large panel of complex patients, hearing the phrase, "Oh, you're a dermatologist too?" when I offer a skin procedure to a patient, has become quite customary. Of course, I explain that I am not a board-certified dermatologist, but when I explain what services I can offer patients within the scope of primary care and procedures I have been trained to do, it provides a broader understanding to the public of the scope of our practices. As one can assume, there are cases when I provide a referral to a subspecialist when medical uncertainty or technical complexity of a proposed procedure dictates a higher level of care and expertise.

Prim Care Clin Office Pract 49 (2022) xi–xii
https://doi.org/10.1016/j.pop.2021.12.003
0095-4543/22/© 2021 Published by Elsevier Inc.

primarycare.theclinics.com

Dermatologic and orthopedic complaints are some of the most common presenting concerns in outpatient primary care practices, and this second consecutive issue of *Primary Care: Clinics in Office Practice* dedicated to office-based procedures highlights various dermatologic and orthopedic procedures. I would like to thank our guest editors, Drs Clebak and Reedy-Cooper, for their exceptional efforts in creating the vision for this issue, and to the authors who wrote very easy-to-follow and comprehensive guides for the procedures highlighted in each article. If you already do some of these procedures, then you can enhance your knowledge with new evidence and improve your skills. If you don't already perform some of these procedures, then consider taking a course or learning from a colleague how to become proficient and credentialed, then expand the services you provide and your joy of the practice of primary care medicine.

Joel J. Heidelbaugh, MD, FAAFP, FACG
Departments of Family Medicine and Urology
University of Michigan Medical School
Ann Arbor, MI, USA

Ypsilanti Health Center
200 Arnet Suite 200
Ypsilanti, MI 48198, USA

E-mail address:
jheidel@umich.edu

Preface

Procedures in Primary Care: Meeting the Comprehensive Needs of Our Patients Where They Are

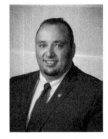   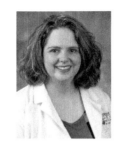

Karl T. Clebak, MD, MHA, FAAFP   Alexis Reedy-Cooper, MD, MPH
Editors

Primary care remains at the front lines in the delivery of patient care. In many of our communities across the United States, patients have limited access to specialty care. Population growth, the aging of the American population, in addition to increased access to care with the Affordable Care Act, have combined to drive the demand for procedural care and highlight the effects of physician shortages.[1] Primary care clinicians have risen to meet this unmet need by continuing to deliver comprehensive care within our communities. The scope of this care has continued to expand and includes a wide variety of office-based procedures across dermatologic, women's health, musculoskeletal, ultrasound, and urgent care.[2] It has also been suggested that family medicine residency programs may need to adjust their training to address specific procedures (ie, the destruction of benign skin lesions, nail care, large joint injection, punch or shave skin biopsy, removal of impacted cerumen, wound debridement, Unna boot application, excision of skin lesion, paring of corn or callus, and insertion of urinary bladder catheter) to better meet the needs of the Medicare patient population.[3]

In this issue, we focus on the procedural care that is routinely provided in the ambulatory care setting, including dermatologic and orthopedic procedures. We review skin biopsy techniques, laceration repair, incision and drainage of abscesses, foreign body removal, cryotherapy, electrosurgery, the treatment of keloids, nail and foot care, dermoscopy, large-, intermediate-, and small-joint injections, tendon and myofascial injections, the management of fractures and sprains, and point-of-care ultrasound for musculoskeletal and other diagnostic applications.

Prim Care Clin Office Pract 49 (2022) xiii–xiv
https://doi.org/10.1016/j.pop.2021.12.002
0095-4543/22/© 2021 Published by Elsevier Inc.

With proper training, incorporating these procedures into your practice can be a fulfilling way to deliver comprehensive care for our patients where they are, in the primary care setting.

Karl T. Clebak, MD, MHA, FAAFP
Department of Family and
Community Medicine
Penn State Health
Milton S. Hershey Medical Center
500 University Drive
Hershey, PA 17033, USA

Alexis Reedy-Cooper, MD, MPH
Department of Family and
Community Medicine
Penn State Health
St. Joseph Medical Center
145 North 6th Street
Reading, PA 19601, USA

E-mail addresses:
Kclebak@pennstatehealth.psu.edu (K.T. Clebak)
areedycooper@pennstatehealth.psu.edu (A. Reedy-Cooper)

REFERENCES

1. Bodenheimer TS, Smith MD. Primary care: proposed solutions to the physician shortage without training more physicians. Health Aff (Millwood) 2013;32(11): 1881–6.
2. Nothnagle M, Sicilia JM, Forman S, et al. Required procedural training in family medicine residency: a consensus statement. Fam Med 2008 Apr;40(4):248–52.
3. Poulin EA, Swartz AW, O'Grady JS, et al. Essential office procedures for Medicare patients in primary care: comparison with family medicine residency training. Fam Med 2019;51(7):574–7.

Skin Biopsy Techniques

Jason D. Greenwood, MD, MS, Stephen P. Merry, MD, MPH,
Christopher L. Boswell, MD*

KEYWORDS

- Skin lesions • Skin cancer • Skin biopsy • Biopsy techniques • Histopathology
- Shave • Punch • Fusiform excisional biopsy

KEY POINTS

- Skin cancers are the most common type of cancer and can be more easily cured if diagnosed early with biopsy.
- Skin biopsies are easy, in-office procedures that can diagnose and treat patients with dermatologic conditions.
- Melanoma and nonmelanoma skin cancers require biopsy for diagnosis to plan definitive treatment.
- Excisional biopsies include saucerization (scoop shave), fusiform, and punch (for lesions able to be encircled). With careful technique, one can excise a whole suspected skin cancer for dermatopathology, removing or destroying additional margins as indicated.
- Punch biopsy is commonly used for full-thickness skin sampling of a larger lesion or rash for diagnosis.

INTRODUCTION

Skin biopsy procedures are essential services for primary care providers to offer to their patients. They can easily be added to the primary care provider's skill set with minimal impact on workflow while improving long-term cosmetic, morbidity, and mortality outcomes. Patients value convenience, so patient satisfaction improves when procedures are offered at the initial visit rather than requiring a return trip. There are also benefits in terms of provider and practice revenue when procedures can be incorporated into visits in real time.[1] A fully stocked procedure cart positioned near examination rooms enables quick and efficient office-based procedures, saving time and frustration when one decides to offer a skin biopsy during a routine clinic visit (**Fig. 1**). Finally, it is useful to have checklists of supplies needed for each procedure you commonly perform available for your staff so they can gather the supplies while you obtain informed consent and prepare the patient.

Skin cancer is the most common form of cancer in the United States,[2] and diagnosis of skin lesions, malignant and benign, is often difficult without biopsy.[3–5] Specialty

Department of Family Medicine, Mayo Clinic, 200 1st Street Southwest, Rochester, MN
55905, USA
* Corresponding author.
E-mail address: Boswell.christopher@mayo.edu

Prim Care Clin Office Pract 49 (2022) 1–22
https://doi.org/10.1016/j.pop.2021.10.001
0095-4543/22/© 2021 Elsevier Inc. All rights reserved.

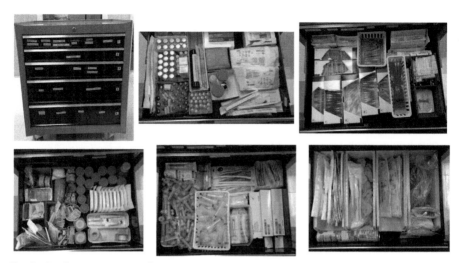

Fig. 1. A primary care procedure cart.

dermatologic services may have limited access in rural areas or long wait times, and primary care providers can avoid delays in diagnosis by performing skin biopsies in their offices.

However, "when in doubt, biopsy" should not be a license for inexperienced clinicians to sample all unknown lesions. Reliable pattern recognition requires study and experience. Additional training in skin lesion identification and dermoscopy is readily available for interested clinicians.[6] For new clinicians, consulting a more experienced colleague by an in-person or a virtual visit may prevent an unnecessary procedure.

DEFINITIONS

Historically, skin biopsy types have caused confusion in nomenclature. Specifically, the term excisional biopsy has most often been used to refer to a traditional, fusiform, full-thickness removal of skin performed with a scalpel. However, punch and saucerization biopsies may also be performed with the intent to excise the entire lesion in question along with a margin of normal surrounding skin. Unfortunately, the Current Procedural Terminology manual, updated in 2019, uses terminology that deemphasizes this point, using the term "tangential" for saucerization biopsies and distinguishing this from punch and "incisional" biopsies.[7] The nuances of each of these types of biopsies have important clinical implications, and medical educators and practitioners should be mindful to use precise language to avoid perpetuating misunderstanding (**Box 1**).

GENERAL INDICATIONS

Skin biopsies are indicated in several clinical scenarios when histopathologic information is required to make a diagnosis and to establish the plan for definitive treatment of the underlying skin condition. The same techniques used for biopsies can also be used for skin and subcutaneous lesion removal even if histopathologic information is not required. Specific indications for the different types of biopsies are detailed later in the procedural techniques section.

Potential indications include the following[8,10]:

- Suspected melanoma or nonmelanoma skin cancer

> **Box 1**
> **Definitions of biopsy types**
>
> Shave biopsy: Partial-thickness (epidermis with or without superficial dermis) biopsy obtained with razor or scalpel with intent to obtain tissue for histopathology and/or remove or reduce the size of a lesion suspected not to be malignant.
>
> Saucerization biopsy: Biopsy performed with razor or scalpel with intent to excise a lesion and margin of surrounding normal skin to the level of the deep dermis.
>
> Punch biopsy: Full-thickness (to the level of subcutaneous fat) biopsy performed with a round or oval-shaped punch tool.
>
> Fusiform excision biopsy: Full-thickness biopsy performed with a scalpel in a fusiform shape.
>
> Subcutaneous nodule biopsy: Complete or partial removal of subcutaneous nodule or lesion with intent to obtain histopathologic diagnosis. Specific techniques exist for certain types of lesions.
>
> *Data from* Refs.[8–11]

- Suspected premalignant skin lesion, such as actinic keratosis, with diagnostic uncertainty
- Difficult-to-diagnose rash
- Blistering skin disorders
- Difficult-to-diagnose or refractory infectious or inflammatory disorder of the skin

GENERAL CONTRAINDICATIONS

Overall, there are few contraindications to skin biopsy.
Potential contraindications include the following[8]:

- Infection
- Excess or supratherapeutic anticoagulation or significant coagulopathy
- Life expectancy
- Sensitive location or large lesion to be biopsied
- Allergy to local anesthetic

If active infection of the biopsy site is of high probability, then treatment of the skin infection should be considered (unless biopsy will play a role in diagnosis). Although anticoagulation is not an absolute contraindication, if bleeding control or hematoma formation after the procedure is a concern, then the proper equipment for treatment needs to be readily available. Life expectancy should be considered, as watchful waiting may be more appropriate than biopsy if no curative procedure is planned after biopsy.[12] Last, anatomic location must be considered. For example, removal of some facial lesions may lead to nerve damage or inability to perform functions, such as fully closing an eye, after wound closure.[13]

ANATOMY
Langer, Wrinkle, and Relaxation Lines

Thoughtful preplanning of the direction and extent of a biopsy will help ensure the best cosmetic outcome and prevent harm. Although Langer lines have historic value, most proceduralists now use relaxed skin tension lines and wrinkle lines, the latter particularly for facial lesions, to plan the orientation of the long axis of an incision or excision.[14] Reviewing one or more anatomic depictions of such lines before a biopsy is helpful (**Fig. 2**), but these lines should be assessed for each patient by gently pinching

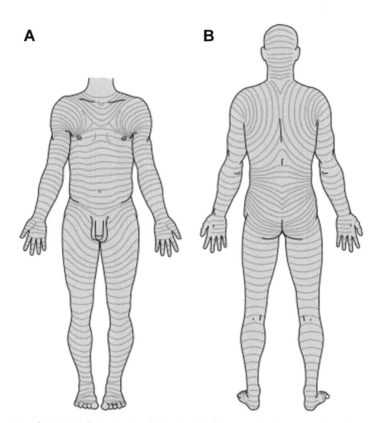

Fig. 2. Lines of minimal skin tension. (*A*) Anterior. (*B*) Posterior. (*From* Sicilia JM. Chapter 18: Incisions: Planning the direction of the incision. In: Fowler GC, ed. Pfenninger and Fowler's Procedures for Primary Care. 4th ed. Elsevier; 2010: 131-135.)

relaxed skin to create a crease when planning a biopsy procedure.[15] Planning for potential scarring to be hidden in a preexisting crease or wrinkle can often achieve better cosmetic outcomes than planning based strictly on an anatomic diagram.

Additional anatomic considerations include vascular and neurologic structures deep to the skin lesion being biopsied and the thickness of the skin (ie, biopsying a lesion on the shin requires a considerably different approach compared with biopsying a lesion on the ear or the back).

SITE SELECTION

Biopsy site selection is important especially if there are multiple lesions. For rashes with multiple stages of healing, lesions roughly 1- to 2-days-old are usually ideal to capture the appropriate change in histopathology. Vesicles should be removed whole, bullae or ulcers need an edge with adequate depth, and large lesions should be sampled at their thickest point with the most variance of color while avoiding necrotic tissue.[9]

GENERAL APPROACH: DECIDING WHAT TO BIOPSY AND HOW

Pattern recognition is important during a clinical skin examination. A review of all the various types of skin lesions is beyond the scope of this article, but it is relevant to discuss a general approach. Notably, current U.S. Preventive Services Task Force (USPSTF) guidelines do not recommend skin cancer screening examinations, citing insufficient evidence,[16] but many questions have been raised about the task force's assessment of the balance of benefits and harms. For example, one multidisciplinary group points out that increasing the detection of basal cell carcinoma may be a benefit rather than a potential harm as described in the USPSTF recommendation statement, and they note that morbidity and financial burden associated with diagnosis of skin cancer at more advanced stages were not considered by the USPSTF.[17]

Certain skin lesions may be readily diagnosed with a quick glance for an experienced provider, whereas others may yield a dramatic surprise upon reading the pathology report. When a benign diagnosis is certain, symptoms related to irritation and cosmetic concerns may be an adequate reason for removal with or without sending the specimen to the pathology laboratory. When a diagnosis is uncertain, the removed specimen should be sent to the pathology laboratory for histopathologic diagnosis. Some institutions have specific guidelines in place such that even obviously benign lesions larger than a certain size are sent for pathologic examination.

Traditionally, pigmented skin lesions are evaluated using the ABCDE criteria, and lesions with Asymmetry, Border irregularities, Colors of concern, Diameter larger than 6 mm, or Evolution or significant growth are recommended for biopsy.[18] In patients with multiple melanocytic nevi, such as those with the atypical nevus syndrome, the ugly duckling sign, identifying a nevus of significantly different morphology than most other nevi on the same type of skin of the same individual, can be a helpful tool.[19] Each of these methods have been used in patient education programs, as well.[20] Recently, dermoscopy has increased in popularity and accessibility for primary care clinicians, and with appropriate training, one can use simple algorithms to improve diagnostic success rates (**Fig. 3**).[21] Artificial intelligence and diagnostic tools that are in development appear to hold great promise for improving sensitivity and specificity of skin cancer diagnosis.[22,23]

The incidence of melanoma has been increasing steadily over the last several decades. There is considerable controversy regarding whether this increase represents a true increase in disease occurrence, whether this increase is a result of increased diagnostic scrutiny related to overzealous biopsy practices, whether there is nonevidence-based skin screening examinations, and whether there are lowered thresholds for pathologists to diagnose microscopic changes as malignant, or a combination of the 2 processes.[24]

For lesions in the epidermis and/or dermis, the 4 biopsy technique options include the following: shave, saucerization, punch, and fusiform excision.[10,11] Most skin lesions encountered and biopsied in the primary care setting are amenable to saucerization, punch, or fusiform excision. Each of these options should be considered with the risks and benefits discussed with the patient. The saucerization technique has several benefits (eg, time needed to perform, absence of required suturing, and acceptable cosmetic outcome with typically mild hypopigmentation or hyperpigmentation), but certain clinical scenarios may necessitate one of the other techniques.[25] For example, diagnosis of a refractory rash or inflammatory skin condition requires full-thickness histopathologic examination, so one or more punch biopsies are usually performed.[26] In locations where the dermis is determined to be too thin to allow for saucerization without high risk of subcutaneous fat herniation and in areas prone to friction, a punch biopsy or a fusiform excision biopsy is required.

Historically, there has been controversy regarding saucerization biopsies of macular pigmented lesions because of concern about the risk of transecting the lesion, which could limit the prognostic value of the biopsy. However, a 2013 study revealed that

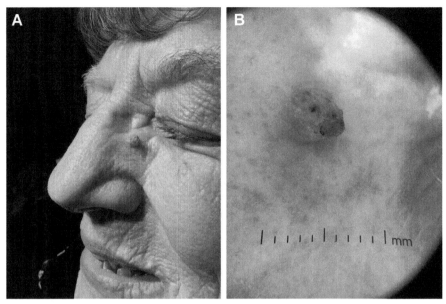

Fig. 3. Comparison of clinical and dermoscopic images of a cutaneous horn arising from squamous cell carcinoma. (*A*) Clinical preoperative image. (*B*) Dermoscopic image.

even though saucerization biopsies resulted in more than twice as many transected melanomas compared with punch biopsy and 6 times as many compared with fusiform excision biopsy, there was no difference in patient survival.[27] It is reasonable to saucerize a lesion for diagnosis even if suspicion is high for a melanoma or a nonmelanoma skin cancer,[28] although some experts would choose a fusiform excision with narrow margins. Reexcision with appropriate margins or destructive procedures (electrodessication [ED&C] or cryotherapy and curettage [C&C]) for nonmelanoma skin cancer can then be performed once the diagnosis is confirmed.[29,30]

STEPS FOR PREPROCEDURE PLANNING

1. Discuss relevant allergies, medical history, medications, and previous experiences with particular attention to bleeding risk.
2. Discuss your plan with the patient, including options for biopsy technique as appropriate.
3. Obtain written or verbal informed consent, depending on your institution's or practice's policies, after discussing risks, benefits, and alternatives of the proposed procedure.
4. Photograph the lesion or lesions to aid future medical decision making.[28]
5. Mark the planned excision path with indelible ink to include the lesion and any margins of normal skin to be removed (**Table 1**). This is important to perform before injection of local anesthetic, which may obscure palpable edges of subcutaneous lesions.

PATIENT POSITIONING AND PREPARATION

1. Position the patient either seated or lying down so that the intended biopsy site is exposed and parallel to the floor, if possible. The procedural team should check

Table 1
Recommended empiric margins for biopsy based on top differential diagnosis

Lesion	Margins, mm[a]	Additional Considerations
Benign lesion	0–2	Obtain 1- to 2-mm margins if diagnosis is not 100% certain
Atypical nevus, rule out melanoma	1–4	Obtain 1- to 2-mm margins regardless of technique if diagnosis is uncertain. Nevi with less than severe atypia with clear histopathologic margins do not require reexcision; nevi with severe atypia require reexcision with 4-mm margins. Melanoma should be referred to a dermatologist for 1- to 3-cm margin-wide excision
Basal or squamous cell carcinoma	1–5	Cure can be achieved at the same time as diagnosis for low-risk lesion subtypes with larger excised margins or through destructive techniques (C&C or ED&C). If the lesion is in the high-risk H-zone of the face (see **Fig. 12**) and will require referral for Mohs surgery once diagnosis is confirmed, 1- to 2-mm margins are most appropriate

[a] Note, these are the authors' recommendations for initial biopsy margins, not definitive surgical treatment that must be individualized and guided by anatomic location and data from the pathology report.

Data from Refs.[9,28,29,30]

with the patient routinely to inquire as to their comfort, as they may need to hold this position for several minutes.
2. Raise the bed to an appropriate height for ergonomics of the proceduralist.
3. Assemble all required and potentially required instruments and medications needed for the biopsy procedure on a tray adjacent to the patient.
4. Perform a timeout or preprocedural pause to ensure the correct procedure will be performed for the correct patient at the correct anatomic location.
5. Double-check your planned pattern of excision or incision to ensure you will be able to approximate your wound edges with your current outline and to confirm the lesion or skin has not shifted during position changes.
6. Consider draping the area with towels or a fenestrated drape to expose the field and minimize body fluid spillage.
7. Don nonsterile gloves; a meta-analysis of multiple studies found no difference in infection rate when sterile versus nonsterile gloves are worn for outpatient dermatologic procedures.[31]

ANESTHESIA

An anesthetic with epinephrine should be used, as it decreases bleeding and prolongs the effect of the anesthetic. Use of epinephrine for anesthesia of the nose, ears, and digits is not only safe without risk of tissue necrosis[32] but also recommended for anesthesia of these highly vascular structures.[33] Allergy to an ester local anesthetic, such as procaine (Novocaine), is not uncommon; it is acceptable in such cases to use lidocaine (Xylocaine) or bupivacaine (Marcaine), which are both amides and for which allergy is uncommon. If the patient is not sure what specific medication they reacted to in the past or are allergic to both amides and esters, intradermal injection of normal saline or subcutaneous 1% diphenhydramine can provide adequate temporary dermal anesthesia.[33] The onset of action of lidocaine and bupivacaine is nearly identical (approximately 5 minutes) injected subcutaneously. Intradermal injection provides immediate anesthesia and is the preferred method for most shave, saucerization, and punch biopsies.

For intradermal injection, use a 27- or 30-g needle, bevel up, positioned superficially under the center of the lesion and inject at a slow rate, to minimize discomfort, to raise a wheal beyond the marked margins to be excised.[34] If multiple injections are required for the same lesion, care should be taken to insert the needle into an area that has already been infiltrated and anesthetized to minimize patient discomfort. A field block is best for a full-thickness lesion removal or subcutaneous nodule biopsy. Inject subcutaneously beyond the edge of any undermining needed to allow for anesthesia while reapproximating wound edges after fusiform excision.

PROCEDURAL APPROACH AND TECHNIQUES
Shave Biopsy

Indications

- Superficial lesions that arise from the epidermis, such as skin tags, warts, and seborrheic keratoses. Pedunculated lesions with narrow-enough stalks can be snipped with scissors rather than using a shave tool as described in later discussion, with or without local anesthetic depending on size and patient preference.
- Lesions that arise from the dermis, such as dermatofibromas and intradermal nevi, which are being removed or transected and shaved flush with surrounding skin for cosmesis reasons or irritation.

Equipment

- Skin marker (**Fig. 4**)
- Paper ruler to measure maximum length of wound
- Syringe (3 mL usually suffices unless multiple lesions are being addressed)
- Needle to draw anesthetic into the syringe (large gauge, such as 18 g)
- Injection needle (small gauge, such as 30 g)
- Local anesthetic of choice with epinephrine
- Alcohol swabs
- Antiseptic preparation solution, swabs, or swab sticks

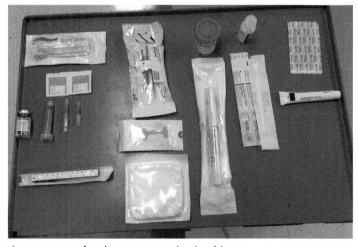

Fig. 4. Equipment set up for shave or saucerization biopsy.

- Double-sided razor or shave biopsy blade (or scalpel or iris scissors if "snip" biopsy is planned)
- Forceps with teeth
- Aluminum chloride with application swabs (or other available hemostatic agent, such as silver nitrate or Monsel solution)
- Petroleum jelly
- Adhesive dressing
- Specimen container with fixation solution
- 4 × 4″ gauze pads
- Thermocautery or electrocautery system (have available but usually not required)

Technique

1. Work surface or tray with all equipment needed and draw up anesthetic.
2. Cleanse the previously demarcated area with an antiseptic preparation.
3. Inject anesthetic intradermally into the lesion to extend just beyond marked border.
4. While applying a slight curve to the blade, use a sawing motion to cut along the planned path either transecting the lesion or just deep to the presumed deep edge of the lesion. Forceps or a cotton-tipped applicator can be used to provide countertraction to the lesion if necessary.
5. If sending the specimen to the pathology laboratory, place the specimen in a properly labeled specimen container.
6. Apply aluminum chloride to the base of the wound to control bleeding and prevent delayed bleeding.
7. Apply petroleum jelly and cover with dressing.

Saucerization Biopsy

Indications

- Suspected nonmelanoma skin cancers with intent to cure or confirm diagnosis before other definitive treatment
- Atypical nevi

Equipment

- All the equipment from the shave biopsy technique (see **Fig. 4**)

Technique

1. Prepare work surface or tray with all equipment needed and draw up anesthetic (**Fig. 5**).
2. Cleanse the previously demarcated area with an antiseptic preparation.
3. Inject anesthesia intradermally into the lesion.
4. Bend the razor or shave biopsy blade and begin excision at one edge with a sawing motion with the blade angled at 30° to 45° to the skin. Raised lesions can be grasped with the forceps and elevated. Continue the sawing motion to the appropriate depth (the goal is to excise to the depth of white to off-white fibrous dermis), relaxing the bend of the blade to follow the demarcated margins, and then gradually adjusting the angle to be parallel to the skin. After passing the center of the lesion, start to angle back upward and bend the blade again to maintain the planned shape of the excision. As you approach the final cuts, it is often helpful to apply countertraction to the skin surface with forceps or cotton-tipped applicator.

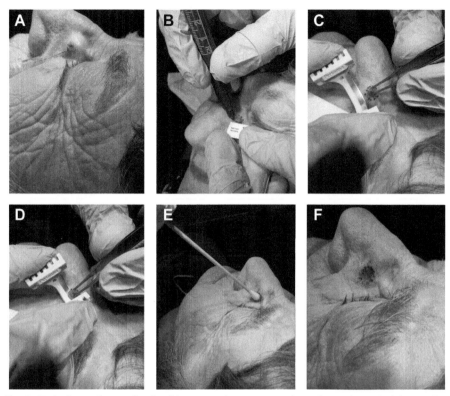

Fig. 5. Technique of saucerization biopsy on the cutaneous horn from Figure 3. (*A*) Intradermal injection of anesthetic. (*B*) Marking 1 mm margins. (*C,D*) Saucerization. (*E*) Application of aluminum chloride for hemostasis. (*F*) Wound will heal by secondary intent.

5. Be sure to excise the entire lesion with adequate depth and at or slightly beyond your demarcated margins. If you notice pigment or lesion remaining in the depth of the wound, reexcise to a subcutaneous fat layer (convert to a fusiform excision).
6. Place the specimen in a properly labeled specimen container.
7. Apply aluminum chloride and/or cautery to the base of the wound to control bleeding and prevent delayed bleeding.
8. Apply petroleum jelly and cover with dressing.

Punch Biopsy

Indications

- Smaller pigmented lesions (generally the largest punch tool is 10 mm, so the lesion must be less than or equal to 6 mm to allow for 2-mm margins)
- Rashes
- Vasculitis
- Bullous diseases (edge of bulla)
- Representative lesions of inflammatory skin disorders
- Very large, pigmented lesions too difficult to biopsy with excisional intent (punch one or more areas of maximal abnormal appearance)

Equipment

- Skin marker (**Fig. 6**)
- Paper ruler to measure maximum length of wound and guide margins
- Syringe (3 mL usually suffices unless multiple lesions are being addressed)
- Needle to draw anesthetic into the syringe (large gauge, such as 18 g)
- Injection needle (small gauge, such as 30 g)
- Local anesthetic of choice with epinephrine
- Alcohol swabs
- Antiseptic preparation solution, swabs, or swab sticks
- Punch biopsy tool (sizes range from 1 mm to 10 mm)
- Forceps with teeth
- Iris scissors
- Needle driver and suture of choice if you intend to close the wound (**Box 2**)
- Aluminum chloride with application swabs (or other available hemostatic agent, such as silver nitrate or Monsel solution)
- Petroleum jelly
- Adhesive dressing
- Specimen container with fixation solution
- 4 × 4″ gauze pads
- Thermocautery or electrocautery system (have available but usually not required)

Technique

1. Prepare work surface or tray with all equipment needed and draw up anesthetic (**Fig. 7**).
2. Cleanse the previously demarcated area with an antiseptic preparation.
3. Inject anesthesia intradermally into and subcutaneously below the lesion.
4. Pinch the surrounding skin to confirm understanding of the skin tension lines and then firmly stretch the skin perpendicular to these lines to result in a more elliptical wound that lies in the skin lines.

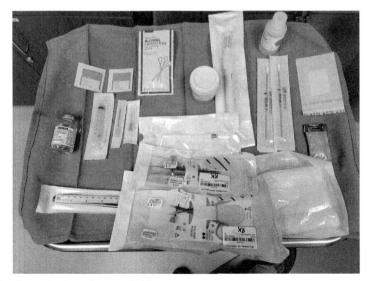

Fig. 6. Equipment set up for punch biopsy.

Box 2
To suture or NOT to suture after punch biopsy

Generally not. Most punch biopsy sites, especially those 4 mm and smaller, and likely all those 8 mm and smaller, heal equally well by secondary intent with acceptable cosmetic results, reducing procedure time and cost over sutured closure. A randomized trial comparing punch biopsy sites closed with suture to sites on the same subject left to heal by secondary intent revealed no significant difference in visual appearance as rated by 3 blinded physicians at 9 months. The subjects were equally satisfied with each method for the 4-mm punches but preferred the appearance of the sutured sites for the 8-mm punches.[35] Another randomized trial comparing purse-string suture to secondary intent healing of circular or oval wounds greater than 8 mm on the trunk and extremities found no significant difference in cosmesis from the patient and 2 blinded observers.[36]

5. Place the punch tool blade against the skin, press lightly, and rotate until you feel the characteristic release as the dermal fascia is cut. Remove the punch tool and release the skin stretching. The island of skin being excised should stand slightly higher than the surrounding skin; this is a signal you have achieved appropriate depth.
6. Elevate the island of skin being excised with forceps or needle and cut the island free from the underlying subcutaneous fat with scissors.
7. Place the specimen in a properly labeled specimen container.
8. Apply aluminum chloride and/or cautery to the base of the wound to control bleeding and prevent delayed bleeding.
9. Apply petroleum jelly and cover with dressing.

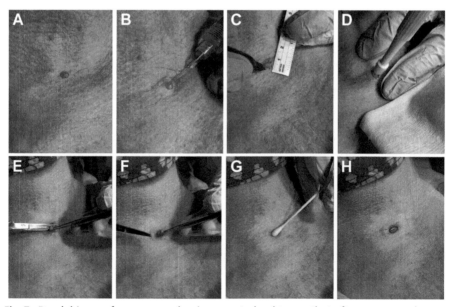

Fig. 7. Punch biopsy of a poroma, a benign sweat gland tumor that often masquerades as a malignant lesion, on the patient's neck. (*A*) Preoperative image. (*B*) Intradermal anesthetic injection. (*C*) Measuring and marking with 1-mm margins. (*D*) Punch incision. (*E, F*) Elevation and excision of the skin island. (*G*) Application of aluminum chloride for hemostasis. (*H*) Wound will heal by secondary intent.

Fusiform Excision Biopsy

Indications

- Very high suspicion for melanoma or high-risk subtype of nonmelanoma skin cancer (morpheaform basal cell carcinoma or invasive squamous cell carcinoma)
- Lesions in anatomic locations less optimal for saucerization (frictional areas)
- Reexcision with appropriate margins of malignant lesions or nevi with severe atypia on initial biopsy
- Any area for which the patient and/or proceduralist opts for a linear scar rather than an area of hypopigmentation or hyperpigmentation that usually results from the techniques described above

Equipment

- Skin marker (**Fig. 8**)
- Paper ruler to measure maximum length of wound and guide margins
- Syringe (5–10 mL usually suffices)
- Needle to draw anesthetic into the syringe (large gauge, such as 18 g)
- Injection needle (small gauge, such as 30 g)
- Local anesthetic of choice with epinephrine
- Alcohol swabs
- Antiseptic preparation solution, swabs, or swab sticks
- Scalpel, typically no. 15 blade or no. 10 blade
- Forceps with teeth
- Curved iris scissors
- Curved hemostat
- Tissue hooks (optional)
- Needle driver and suture of choice, usually absorbable and nonabsorbable
- Adhesive dressing or materials for a wrap-style pressure dressing, depending on location
- Specimen container with fixation solution

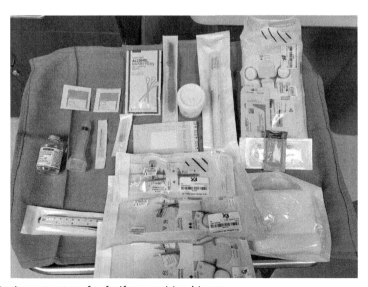

Fig. 8. Equipment set up for fusiform excision biopsy.

- 4 × 4″ gauze pads
- Thermocautery or electrocautery system (have available but usually not required)

Technique

1. Prepare work surface or tray with all equipment needed and draw up anesthetic (**Fig. 9**).
2. Cleanse the previously demarcated area with an antiseptic preparation.
   a. The planned excision should be approximately 3:1 length:width dimensions, which leaves at least a 30° angle at each corner (**Fig. 10**).
   b. Mark both the planned excision lines and the area of planned undermining (undermine on each side at the top of the fat layer a width of tissue, which is the same as the width of the planned excision at that point).
3. Inject anesthesia intradermally along the planned excision lines as well as a field block to the edge of the demarcated area of planned undermining.
4. While applying countertraction with the nondominant hand, start at one corner and use the scalpel to cut along one side of the planned excision at the appropriate depth. Keep the blade perpendicular to the skin or blade angled away from the lesion to achieve eversion of the wound edges when closed (**Fig. 11**).
5. While applying countertraction with the nondominant hand, start at the same first corner and cut along the other side of the planned excision at the same depth. Carry the incision down to the yellow subcutaneous fat layer.
6. Elevate the island of skin being excised with forceps or needle and cut the island free from the underlying subcutaneous fat with scissors or scalpel. The best practice is to elevate one end and dissect from that end to the midpoint and then repeat from the other end; it is easy to dissect too deeply if you dissect in the same direction all the way along the full length of the excision.
7. Tag the specimen with a suture at one corner and indicate its orientation in the pathology order. Place the specimen in a properly labeled specimen container.
8. Control any brisk bleeding with pressure, cautery, and/or a figure-of-eight absorbable suture.
9. Lift the edges of the wound with forceps or tissue hook and undermine in the plane between the subcutaneous fat and the dermis to mobilize the skin and allow low-tension closure.
10. Close the wound in an intermediate layered fashion first with buried absorbable sutures (the practice "deep to superficial, superficial to deep" allows for the knot to be buried) and then close the epidermis with simple interrupted, running, or mattress sutures, Steri-Strips, or skin glue. Epidermal "top" sutures should reapproximate, not strangulate, the skin at the wound edges. Strive to leave the wound edges everted.
11. Apply appropriate dressing to cover; consider a pressure dressing.

Subcutaneous Nodule Biopsy: Lipoma

Indications

- A lipoma that is bothersome to the patient or a subcutaneous nodule concerning to the provider. Point of care or formal ultrasound can be a helpful preprocedural diagnostic tool and has been shown to improve provider confidence in performing other dermatologic procedures, such as abscess incision and drainage.[35]

Equipment

- All the equipment from the Fusiform Excision Biopsy technique

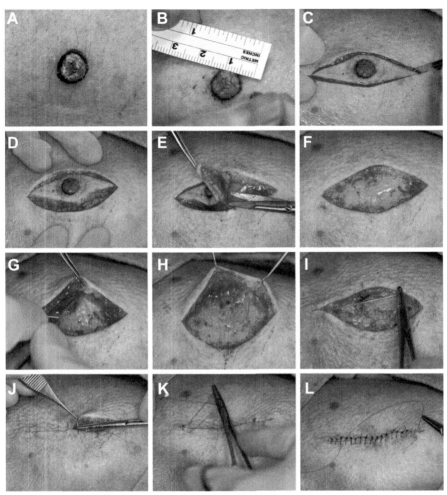

Fig. 9. Fusiform excision of a squamous cell carcinoma. (*A, B*) After the lesion and appropriate margins are marked, the site is anesthetized, prepared with an antiseptic agent, and draped with sterile towels. (*C*) Stabilizing the site with traction, the epidermis on one side of the fusiform design is scored using a no. 15 blade, and then the opposite side is scored. (*D*) The incision is completed into the appropriate plane in the subcutaneous tissue, and the specimen then sits up in the middle of the wound, like an island. (*E, F*) The base of the specimen is dissected with scissors or a blade. (*G, H*) The wound edges are then undermined in the same plane as the base of the wound with blunt-tipped scissors or a blade. Electrodesiccation or electrocoagulation is used to address small actively bleeding vessels to achieve hemostasis. (*I, J*) The subepidermal space is closed with buried sutures. (*K, L*) The epidermal edges are opposed by simple interrupted sutures. (*From* Olbricht S. Chapter 146: Biopsy techniques and basic excisions. In: Bolognia JL, Schaffer JV, Cerroni L, eds. Dermatology. 4th ed. Elsevier; 2018: 2478-2494.)

Technique

1. work surface or tray with all the equipment needed and draw up the anesthetic.
2. Cleanse the previously demarcated area with an antiseptic preparation.

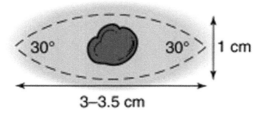

Fig. 10. Creating an ellipse (proper dimensions). (*From* Sicilia JM. Chapter 18: Incisions: Planning the direction of the incision. In: Fowler GC, ed. Pfenninger and Fowler's Procedures for Primary Care. 4th ed. Elsevier; 2010: 131-135.)

     a. A linear incision over the top of the lipoma (length at least half the length of the palpated lesion) is all that is required, but for superficial lesions that have stretched the skin such that the overlying skin appears irreversibly altered, removing enough skin in a fusiform fashion that the postoperative skin will lie flat is advised.

     b. Mark the planned incision lines. No undermining should be needed.

3. Inject anesthesia intradermally along the planned incision and subcutaneously in a field block. Grasp and lift the lipoma from the underlying tissues, and if accessible and safe, inject a few milliliters under the lesion as well.

4. While applying countertraction with the nondominant hand, incise through the dermis to the level of subcutaneous fat or the edge of the lipoma capsule.

5. Develop the plane between dermis and lipoma using a curved hemostat, spinning the open hemostat tips 360° to free the lesion from surrounding tissues.

6. Firmly squeeze the sides of the lesion, as some lipomas will be minimally adherent and readily expressed. Continue to use blunt and sharp dissection to free the lesion from the surrounding tissue. Keep in mind that a minority of lipomas are

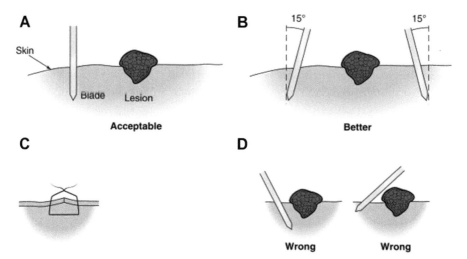

Fig. 11. The proper angle of the scalpel when creating an ellipse. (*A*) Acceptable angle. (*B*) Better angle. (*C*) Proper shapes of suture and skin margins on completion of closure. (*D*) Wrong angles. (*From* Sicilia JM. Chapter 18: Incisions: Planning the direction of the incision. In: Fowler GC, ed. Pfenninger and Fowler's Procedures for Primary Care. 4th ed. Elsevier; 2010: 131-135.)

encapsulated, so distinguishing the abnormal fatty, lesion tissue from normal surrounding subcutaneous fat can be challenging. Any loosely adherent, morphologically large globules should be considered part of the lesion and removed. Irrigation or gentle curettage of the walls can help reveal additional loosely adherent tissue.

7. Gross examination of the lesion may aid decisions for pathologic examination. Place the specimen in a properly labeled specimen container for pathologic analysis.
8. Control any brisk bleeding with pressure, cautery, and/or figure-of-eight suture with absorbable suture.
9. If a significant defect is created by removal of the subcutaneous lesion, use absorbable sutures to close the deep space to reduce risk of seroma formation.
10. Close the wound, often in an intermediate layered fashion first with buried absorbable sutures and then the epidermis with simple interrupted, running, or mattress sutures, Steri-Strips, or skin glue. The layer of epidermal "top" sutures should reapproximate, not strangulate, the skin at the wound edges. Strive to leave the wound edges everted with the corners flat.
11. Apply appropriate dressing to cover; consider a pressure dressing.

Subcutaneous Nodule Biopsy: Epidermoid cyst

Indications

- Epidermoid, sebaceous, or pilar cysts. Point-of-care ultrasound can be a valuable diagnostic tool to ensure the lesion is a fluid-filled structure (hypoechoic with posterior acoustic enhancement).

Equipment

- All the equipment from fusiform excision biopsy, plus the following:
  - Punch biopsy tool (3-5 mm, optional for a variation on the minimal incision technique)
  - 11 blade may be substituted for the no. 10 or 15 blade scalpel

Technique

1. work surface or tray with all equipment needed and draw up the anesthetic.
2. Cleanse the previously demarcated area with an antiseptic preparation.
   a. For this technique, often a linear incision over the top of the cyst (length at least half the length of the palpated lesion) is all that is required, but for superficial lesions that have stretched the skin, such that the overlying skin appears irreversibly altered, removing most or all the abnormal skin in a fusiform fashion is advised. Also, consider a very narrow fusiform excision to remove the enlarged pore, which is an often encountered finding in this type of lesion.
   b. This section describes excision of the encapsulated cyst with commonly required adjustments, but an alternative method called the minimal incision technique is well described and often provides excellent results or a hybrid method becomes necessary when the cyst wall ruptures during attempted removal in toto. This method involves a 3- to 4-mm incision (or punch) over and into the cyst, evacuation of the contents, and piecemeal removal of the cyst wall. Frequently, no closure is required.[36]
3. Inject anesthesia intradermally along the planned incision and in a field block. Eye and clothing protection is imperative, as inadvertent injection into the cyst can cause pressurized spatter of anesthetic and cyst contents.

4. While applying countertraction with the nondominant hand, cut along the planned incision or excision line or lines through the dermis to the level of the superficial cyst wall.
5. Carefully dissect the capsule free of the surrounding tissue. This can be challenging if the cyst has been inflamed previously; if the cyst ruptures, grieve but do not despair.
6. Whether piecemeal or in toto, ensure removal of as much of the cyst wall as possible. Irrigation or gentle curettage or swabbing of the wound walls can help reveal additional pieces of cyst contents or wall.
7. If there is any concern for a diagnosis other than simple inclusion cyst, place the specimen or specimens in a properly labeled specimen container.
8. Control any brisk bleeding with cautery and pressure or figure-of-eight suture with absorbable suture.
9. If a significant defect is created by removal of the subcutaneous lesion, use absorbable sutures to close the deep space to reduce risk of seroma and abscess formation.
10. Close the wound, often in an intermediate layered fashion, first with buried absorbable sutures, and then the epidermis with simple interrupted, running, or mattress sutures, Steri-Strips, or skin glue. Epidermal "top" sutures should reapproximate, not strangulate, the skin at the wound edges. Strive to leave the wound edges everted with the corners flat.
11. Apply appropriate dressing to cover; consider a pressure dressing.

RECOVERY AND PATIENT POSTPROCEDURE INSTRUCTIONS

The dressing should be left in place overnight, and typically showering the following day is acceptable. The wound should be kept clean and dry, and any wound healing by secondary intent can be treated with petroleum jelly until healed.

If sutures are to be removed, instruct the patient on appropriate timing (**Box 3**). At the time of suture removal, if there is concern for dehiscence because of tension, then Steri-Strips can be applied to provide additional strength for 7 days.

COMPLICATIONS
Biopsy Site Infection

During wound healing, there may be some slight increasing redness around the biopsy site. If there is some concern for possible early infection, treatment with dilute vinegar (50:50 vinegar to water) 3 times a day for 5 days is an option when close follow-up is

---

Box 3
Approximate number of days for sutures to remain in place

- Face: 4 to 7
- Scalp and neck: 7 to 14
- Trunk: 10 to 14
- Upper extremity: 7 to 10
- Lower extremity: 10 to 14
- Palms and soles: 14 to 21

Data from Refs.[9,10,37]

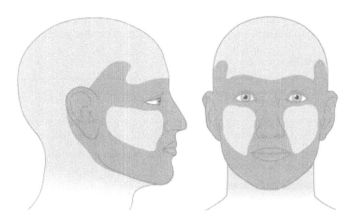

Fig. 12. H-zone of the face. (*From* James WD, Elston DM, Treat JR, Rosenbach MA, Neuhaus IM. Dermatologic Surgery. In: James WD, Elston DM, Treat JR, Rosenbach MA, Neuhaus IM, eds. Andrews' Diseases of the Skin. 13 ed. E-Book: Elsevier; 2019:881-908.)

available. If erythema spreads or streaks, purulent drainage is noted, or systemic symptoms or signs develop, then oral antibiotics may be needed with empiric coverage for common skin pathogens. Lesions that have been closed with sutures may require early suture removal to allow drainage of purulent material.

Bleeding

Delayed bleeding rarely complicates skin biopsies. Patients should be instructed to return for reevaluation for bleeding that does not stop after 15 minutes of direct pressure.

FOLLOW-UP

It is important to develop a working relationship with your dermatopathology team. The pathology report guides definitive treatment planning for the patient for whom the biopsy was performed, but it can also provide valuable information that helps the proceduralist adjust their technique and develop their lesion identification skills over time.

Malignant lesions require additional treatment after biopsy. Depending on the diagnosis, this could include reexcision, referral to a dermatologic surgeon for Mohs micrographic surgery, or destructive methods, such as C&C or ED&C. In certain circumstances, it is appropriate to apply such destructive methods to the wound base immediately following initial biopsy. For example, a small lesion highly suspicious for nonmelanoma skin cancer on the trunk or extremities of an older patient can be treated with C&C or ED&C, saving the patient from a return trip and second procedure when the pathology report confirms the initial suspicion. This treatment option should not be offered if the lesion is removed from the high-risk H-zone of the face (**Fig. 12**).[38] Watchful waiting, rather than any definitive treatment, may be appropriate in patients with limited life expectancy owing to age or medical comorbidities.[12]

SUMMARY

Skin biopsies performed in a primary care clinic can provide patients with diagnosis and treatment without the need for specialist referral. They are useful procedures for the primary care clinician and are appropriate for the outpatient clinical setting. Good technique can minimize scarring and optimize cosmetic outcomes.

CLINICS CARE POINTS

- Plan the extent, orientation, and margins of a biopsy carefully in order to achieve the best cosmetic result.
- Most lesions requiring biopsy in a primary care setting can be biopsied with the saucerization technique, which is fast, requires no repair, and typically has an excellent cosmetic outcome.
- Fusiform excisions are indicated when a linear scar is preferred over an ovoid scar and in areas that are not amenable to saucerization.
- Punch biopsy sites generally do not require suture repair.

DISCLOSURE

The authors have nothing to disclose.

REFERENCES

1. Martz WD. How to boost your bottom line with an office procedure. Fam Pract Manag 2003;10(10):38–40.
2. What is skin cancer? Center for Disease Control. Published 2020. https://www.cdc.gov/cancer/skin/basic_info/what-is-skin-cancer.htm. Accessed July 14, 2020.
3. Ek EW, Giorlando F, Su SY, et al. Clinical diagnosis of skin tumours: how good are we? ANZ J Surg 2005;75(6):415–20.
4. Heal CF, Raasch BA, Buettner PG, et al. Accuracy of clinical diagnosis of skin lesions. Br J Dermatol 2008;159(3):661–8.
5. Shenenberger DW. Cutaneous malignant melanoma: a primary care perspective. Am Fam Physician 2012;85(2):161–8.
6. Dinnes J, Deeks JJ, Chuchu N, et al. Dermoscopy, with and without visual inspection, for diagnosing melanoma in adults. Cochrane Database Syst Rev 2018;12: CD011902.
7. Nicoletti B. Skin deep: how to properly code for biopsies and lesion removal. Fam Pract Manag 2019;26(2):15–9.
8. Pfenninger JL. Skin biopsy. In: Pfenninger JL, Fowler GC, editors. Pfenninger and Fowler's procedures for primary care. 4th edition. E-Book: Elsevier Health Sciences:Philadelphia, PA; 2010. p. 179–85.
9. Olbricht S. Biopsy techniques and basic excisions. In: Bolognia JL, Schaffer JV, Cerroni L, editors. Dermatology. 4th edition. Philadelphia: Elsevier Saunders; 2018. p. 2478–94.
10. Pickett H. Shave and punch biopsy for skin lesions. Am Fam Physician 2011; 84(9):995–1002.
11. Nischal U, Nischal K, Khopkar U. Techniques of skin biopsy and practical considerations. J Cutan Aesthet Surg 2008;1(2):107–11.
12. Chauhan R, Munger BN, Chu MW, et al. Age at diagnosis as a relative contraindication for intervention in facial nonmelanoma skin cancer. JAMA Surg 2018; 153(4):390–2.
13. Alguire PC, Mathes BM. Skin biopsy techniques for the internist. J Gen Intern Med 1998;13(1):46–54.

14. Carmichael SW. The tangled web of Langer's lines. Clin Anat 2014;27(2):162–8.
15. Sicilia JM. Incisions: planning the direction of the incision. In: Pfenninger JL, Fowler GC, editors. Pfenninger and Fowler's procedures for primary care. 4th edition. E-Book: Elsevier Health Sciences:Philadelphia, PA; 2010. p. 131–5.
16. USPST Force, Bibbins-Domingo K, Grossman DC, et al. Screening for skin cancer: US Preventive Services Task Force Recommendation Statement. JAMA 2016;316(4):429–35.
17. Johnson MM, Leachman SA, Aspinwall LG, et al. Skin cancer screening: recommendations for data-driven screening guidelines and a review of the US Preventive Services Task Force controversy. Melanoma Manag 2017;4(1):13–37.
18. American Academy of Dermatology Ad Hoc Task Force for the AoM, Tsao H, Olazagasti JM, Cordoro KM, et al. Early detection of melanoma: reviewing the ABCDEs. J Am Acad Dermatol 2015;72(4):717–23.
19. Gaudy-Marqueste C, Wazaefi Y, Bruneu Y, et al. Ugly duckling sign as a major factor of efficiency in melanoma detection. JAMA Dermatol 2017;153(4):279–84.
20. Ilyas M, Costello CM, Zhang N, et al. The role of the ugly duckling sign in patient education. J Am Acad Dermatol 2017;77(6):1088–95.
21. Rogers T, Marino ML, Dusza SW, et al. A clinical aid for detecting skin cancer: the Triage Amalgamated Dermoscopic Algorithm (TADA). J Am Board Fam Med 2016;29(6):694–701.
22. Tschandl P, Rinner C, Apalla Z, et al. Human-computer collaboration for skin cancer recognition. Nat Med 2020;26(8):1229–34.
23. Du-Harpur X, Watt FM, Luscombe NM, et al. What is AI? Applications of artificial intelligence to dermatology. Br J Dermatol 2020;183(3):423–30.
24. Welch HG, Mazer BL, Adamson AS. The rapid rise in cutaneous melanoma diagnoses. N Engl J Med 2021;384(1):72–9.
25. Gambichler T, Senger E, Rapp S, et al. Deep shave excision of macular melanocytic nevi with the razor blade biopsy technique. Dermatol Surg 2000;26(7):662–6.
26. Sina B, Kao GF, Deng AC, et al. Skin biopsy for inflammatory and common neoplastic skin diseases: optimum time, best location and preferred techniques. A critical review. J Cutan Pathol 2009;36(5):505–10.
27. Mir M, Chan CS, Khan F, et al. The rate of melanoma transection with various biopsy techniques and the influence of tumor transection on patient survival. J Am Acad Dermatol 2013;68(3):452–8.
28. Swetter SM, Tsao H, Bichakjian CK, et al. Guidelines of care for the management of primary cutaneous melanoma. J Am Acad Dermatol 2019;80(1):208–50.
29. Work G, Invited R, Kim JYS, et al. Guidelines of care for the management of basal cell carcinoma. J Am Acad Dermatol 2018;78(3):540–59.
30. Work G, Invited R, Kim JYS, et al. Guidelines of care for the management of cutaneous squamous cell carcinoma. J Am Acad Dermatol 2018;78(3):560–78.
31. Brewer JD, Gonzalez AB, Baum CL, et al. Comparison of sterile vs nonsterile gloves in cutaneous surgery and common outpatient dental procedures: a systematic review and meta-analysis. JAMA Dermatol 2016;152(9):1008–14.
32. Ilicki J. Safety of epinephrine in digital nerve blocks: a literature review. J Emerg Med 2015;49(5):799–809.
33. Kouba DJ, LoPiccolo MC, Alam M, et al. Guidelines for the use of local anesthesia in office-based dermatologic surgery. J Am Acad Dermatol 2016;74(6):1201–19.
34. Scarfone RJ, Jasani M, Gracely EJ. Pain of local anesthetics: rate of administration and buffering. Ann Emerg Med 1998;31(1):36–40.

35. Greenlund LJS, Merry SP, Thacher TD, et al. Primary care management of skin abscesses guided by ultrasound. Am J Med 2017;130(5):e191-3.
36. Zuber TJ. Minimal excision technique for epidermoid (sebaceous) cysts. Am Fam Physician 2002;65(7):1409–12, 1417-1408, 1420.
37. Usatine RP, Coates WC. Laceration and incision repair. In: Pfenninger JL, Fowler GC, editors. Pfenninger and Fowler's procedures for primary care. 4th edition. E-Book: Elsevier Health Sciences:Philadelphia, PA; 2010. p. 136–48.
38. James WD, Elston DM, Treat JR, et al. Dermatologic surgery. In: James WD, Elston DM, Treat JR, et al, editors. Andrews' diseases of the skin. 13th edition. E-Book: Elsevier; 2019. p. 881–908.

A Stitch in Time
Operative and Nonoperative
Laceration Repair Techniques

Benjamin Silverberg, MD, MSc[a,b,c,]*, Amy Moyers, MD[b],
Benjamin I. Wainblat, MD[d], Peter Cashio, MD, MS[e,f],
Kevin Bernstein, MD, MMS, CAQSM[g]

KEYWORDS

- Laceration • Mechanism of injury • Antibiotic prophylaxis • Tissue adhesive
- Staples • Local anesthesia • Scar minimization • Complications

KEY POINTS

- The type of laceration repair performed depends on several factors, including what caused the injury, where and how deep it is, and when the patient presented for treatment.
- A standardized approach to wound repair may avoid missed steps (eg, neglecting to irrigate the wound) and improve the speed at which the patient can be evaluated and treated.
- The most common options for primary laceration repair in an ambulatory clinic include traditional sutures, tissue glues, adhesive strips, staples, and novel techniques such as hair apposition.
- In some situations (eg, animal bites not in so-called critical areas), wounds can be permitted to heal by secondary intention, although prophylactic antibiotics may be necessary.

GENERAL PRINCIPLES OF LACERATION REPAIR

The mechanism of injury, depth and location of wound, involvement of nearby structures, and the length of time elapsed since the injury should be considered when first evaluating a patient presenting with lacerations and/or puncture wounds. Laceration

[a] Department of Emergency Medicine, WVU Medicine, 1 Medical Center Drive, Box 9149, Morgantown, WV 26505, USA; [b] Department of Family Medicine, WVU Medicine, 6040 University Town Center Drive, Morgantown, WV 26501, USA; [c] Division of Physician Assistant Studies, Department of Human Performance, West Virginia University School of Medicine, 64 Medical Center Drive, Box 9226, Morgantown, WV 26505, USA; [d] Department of Family and Community Health, Marshall University Joan C. Edwards School of Medicine, 1600 Medical Center Drive, Huntington, WV 25701, USA; [e] Code 1 Concierge Care, 14101 US 290, Suite 400B, Austin, TX 78737, USA; [f] Baptist Emergency Hospital, 16977 I-35 North, Schertz, TX 78154, USA; [g] Department of Orthopedics and Sports Medicine, United States Naval Academy, 6th Wing, Bancroft Hall, Annapolis, MD 21402, USA
* Corresponding author. WVU Student Health, 390 Birch Street, Morgantown, WV 26506, USA.
E-mail address: benjamin.silverberg@hsc.wvu.edu

Prim Care Clin Office Pract 49 (2022) 23–38
https://doi.org/10.1016/j.pop.2021.10.008
0095-4543/22/© 2021 Elsevier Inc. All rights reserved.
primarycare.theclinics.com

repair should be appropriately triaged in the patient's overall clinical presentation. (For instance, was the head wound sustained in an assault or from a syncopal episode resulting in a fall? If the wound does not require urgent surgical intervention, other pressing medical concerns may need to be addressed first.) Further, the age of the patient, their ability to cooperate during the evaluation and repair, and their expectations for the outcome can further dictate the type of intervention offered.

Initial Wound Evaluation

Visual inspection and gentle irrigation of the wound should be performed, even if there is no obvious foreign debris. The goal of wound irrigation is to dilute the wound's bacterial load; this is best achieved with approximately 50 to 100 cc of irrigation solution per centimeter of wound length. A 35 cc syringe with a 19-gauge needle can be used for more focused cleansing and to better estimate the applied volume. A wound measuring 5 cm, for example, would require at least 250 cc of water for irrigation.[1] Plain, potable water may be preferable to dilute iodine, as the latter can be irritating to raw tissue. In addition, multiple studies have shown that sterile saline is no more efficacious compared with tap water.[1–5] Warmed irrigation solution may be more comfortable for the patient.[6] Avoid being too aggressive when washing a wound; irrigation under pressure can actually force contaminants deeper. (To be sure, the optimal pressure for irrigation is about 5–8 PSI.) Active irrigation is thought to be superior to soaking the affected area, as pruning of the skin from prolonged immersion can make repair more difficult and lead to suboptimal wound closure.[3] Some investigators have suggested soaking may also increase risk of infection.[7,8]

The evaluating clinician should consider if the injury damaged nearby vessels, nerves, soft tissue, or bone. Stanching any bleeding can prevent formation of hematomas and allow for deeper inspection of the wound. Specialist consultation should be obtained when the injury includes open fractures, neurologic deficit, or otherwise suggests the need for more advanced care, as listed in **Box 1**.

If the wound is caused or contaminated by foreign debris such as dirt, metal pieces, or glass, which is not immediately visible to the clinician, then plain radiographs,

---

Box 1
Indications for specialist (surgical) consultation for wound repair

Open fractures (the bone does not need to have broken the skin to be considered "open"), including severe crush injuries

Nerve injury with impaired function

Laceration involving an artery or joint and/or leading to vascular compromise

Involvement of tendons and/or muscles in the hands or feet

Laceration of the salivary duct or canaliculus

Laceration of the eye or eyelid deeper than the subcutaneous layer

Injuries requiring sedation for repair

Severely contaminated wounds that would require long-term drain placement

Strong personal or parental concern for cosmetic outcomes

Other injuries beyond the clinician's scope or level of comfort

---

Data from Refs.[1,7]

ultrasound, and/or computerized tomography (CT) scanning may be appropriate, depending on the size and location of the laceration and available resources. Up to one-third of foreign objects may be missed on initial wound evaluation.[1] Though some debate still exists, both leaded and nonleaded glass fragments as small as 0.5mm should be visible on plain x-rays.[9]

In addition to the wound depth, quality (eg, jagged edges, avulsed skin), and body location, the amount of time since the injury should be considered when determining appropriate repair. Primary closure may occur up to 18 hours after injury (24 hours for wounds of the head).[1] Factors that increase the likelihood of wound infection include contamination, length (>5 cm), location (the lower extremities), and comorbidities (eg, diabetes mellitus).[1,7]

Debridement

Devitalized and necrotic tissue should be removed to reduce the risk of wound infection.[1] However, wounds involving the face should be debrided conservatively, as removing subcutaneous fat may lead to depression of subsequent scars.[1] Further, if small flaps of skin are left in place to better protect the wound, the patient should be cautioned that the tissue will eventually slough off.

Wound Prophylaxis

Tetanus immunization status should be verified with the patient or caregiver. Routine DTaP (diphtheria, tetanus, and acellular pertussis) vaccination begins at 2 months of age, with 3 of the 5 required doses given by 6 months of age. DTaP is given to children younger than 7 years; Tdap is preferred thereafter, ideally with a dose at age 11 to 12 years. Booster shots (Tdap or Td) are given every 10 years.[10]

Patients presenting with lacerations who are also pregnant and patients who have received fewer than 3 doses of tetanus toxoid should receive a dose of Tdap at the time of service. For clean, minor wounds, previously immunized patients should receive a booster only if 10 years or more have elapsed since their last dose. If the wound is contaminated (eg, involving dirt, soil, feces, and/or saliva) or results from a higher-risk mechanism (eg, puncture, shrapnel, avulsion, crush, thermal injury), a booster is appropriate if 5 years or more have passed since the last tetanus toxoid–containing vaccine dose. Tetanus immune globulin is only necessary for patients with contaminated wounds who also never received more than or equal to 3 doses of tetanus vaccine or who have human immunodeficiency virus or severe immunodeficiency (even if the wound is thought to be minor).[7,10-12]

Topical antibiotics (eg, bacitracin zinc) may be considered both for their antimicrobial indication but also as a physical impediment to introduction of other bacteria to the wound.[13] Such ointments should not be used with dissolvable sutures, and care should be taken with triple antibiotic ointment (neomycin, bacitracin, and polymyxin), as some people develop a localized reaction to it, misinterpreting that as infection.

Prophylactic oral or parenteral antibiotics may also be needed if the wound is visibly soiled or contaminated, due to an animal or human bite, or in a high-risk part of the body. Before prescribing, always ensure adjustment of dosage for renal function and use an available local or institutional antibiogram for optimization of microbial coverage. For healthy patients with uncomplicated traumatic skin lacerations, no prophylactic antibiotics are indicated. However, they should be cautioned to seek reevaluation should signs of infection develop, such as fever or localized pain, erythema, swelling, or purulent drainage.[14]

Appropriate empirical antibiotics following water exposure include levofloxacin and either a first-generation cephalosporin (eg, cephalexin, cefazolin) or clindamycin.

Doxycycline should be added for coverage of *Vibrio* species if the wound was exposed to seawater. If the wound has been exposed to soil- or sewage-contaminated water, metronidazole should be added for anaerobic coverage, unless clindamycin has already been used.[15,16] Penetrating injuries through the sole of a shoe or sandal should be treated with antibiotics active against *Pseudomonas* (eg, cipro-floxacin, levofloxacin).

Prophylactic antibiotics for an animal bite wound are given for 3 to 5 days or longer but are not indicated for human bites that do not break the skin or are very superfi-cial.[17] In this setting, cephalexin, dicloxacillin, and erythromycin should be avoided due to lack of activity against *Pasteurella multocida* and *Eikenella corrodens*.[14]

Some investigators have suggested that uncomplicated dog bites may be sutured with improved cosmesis and no worse rate of infection.[1,18,19] Cat bite injuries, on the other hand, should be irrigated but allowed to close by secondary intention unless the wound is on the face.[1] In some cases, loose application of wound adhesive strips can be used to approximate the wound edges.

Postexposure prophylaxis against rabies should be offered for mammalian bites in endemic areas, especially if the injury was not provoked, the animal could not be captured for observation, or the animal's vaccination status is unknown.

QUASI-OPERATIVE TECHNIQUES

Although suturing is the mainstay for laceration repair, many comparable and accept-able options for repair are available depending on the laceration or wound character-istics such as cause and location, as well as patient demographics. Tissue adhesives, wound adhesive strips, stapling, hair apposition technique (HAT), and secondary intention healing are a few of those alternative methods.

Tissue Adhesives (Cyanoacrylates)

Two types of tissue adhesive are available in the United States, n-butyl-2-cyanoacry-late (brand-names: Histoacryl Blue, Periacryl) and 2-octyl-cyanoacrylate (brand-names: Dermabond, Surgiseal).[1] Tissue adhesives are comparable with sutures for closing skin wounds regarding wound infection, wound dehiscence, cosmesis, and patient acceptance.[20-22] Tissue adhesives are also cost-effective compared with su-tures, as they require less application time and do not require return appointments for removal.[1]

To apply tissue adhesive, the wound's edges are approximated, and semi-viscous adhesive liquid is applied in a thin layer over laceration with a 5 mm overlap on each side. Three to four layers are then applied with 30 seconds between applications for the preceding layer to dry. Full tensile strength is achieved after 2.5 minutes.[21] Pediatric patients should be warned of a slight exothermic reaction as the adhesive dries. Many tissue glues have a slight hue to facilitate application; the adhesive turns clear when dry.

To remove misapplied tissue adhesive, wipe it off quickly with dry gauze. If the ad-hesive has dried, apply petroleum-based ointment for 30 minutes and then wipe away.[1] Tissue adhesives are most effective in low-tension skin areas for the repair of clean, simple, and small hemostatic lacerations. They should not be used on lacer-ations that are older than 12 hours; contaminated, infected, or devitalized; located in a mucocutaneous junction; located in a high-tension area; located in a moisture-rich area (eg, groin, axillae); located between the eyebrow and the eye itself; result from a mammalian bite; or have any concern for infection or impaired wound healing due to the patient's chronic conditions.[1,21]

Tissue adhesives form a protective barrier promoting wound healing with potential antimicrobial effects and will slough off spontaneously in 5 to 10 days. For postrepair care, it is important to remind patients not to use petroleum-based ointments for scar minimization, as this can remove the tissue adhesive before the wound is healed.[21] Overall, tissue adhesives allow timely laceration repair with minimal pain, making them a great choice for pediatric patients.

Wound Adhesive Strips

Wound adhesive strips (brand-name Steri-Strips) are also used to approximate clean, simple, and small lacerations located in areas of low skin tension and are not bleeding.[1] They have been found to have the same cosmetic outcomes as tissue adhesive; however, they do lack tensile strength and may cause local inflammatory reactions from the adhesives that can lead to wound dehiscence.[1,21] Wound adhesive strips are applied perpendicular to the wound in a manner that will approximate the wound edges.[1] The indications and benefits for wound adhesive strips are the same as those for tissue adhesives.

Stapling

Staples are faster and more cost-effective than sutures with no difference in complications. Staples create a loose closure of the wound edges allowing for drainage and making them the appropriate technique for unclean wounds if needed.[1] Staples are recommended for closure of thick skin on the extremities, trunk, and scalp (where hair can make both placement and removal of sutures difficult) but not on the face, neck, hands, or feet.[21] Staples are applied perpendicular to the wound. Ready access to a staple remover during the procedure for potential misfires or incorrect placement is recommended. Furthermore, be sure to avoid placement of stainless-steel staples for scalp wounds if CT or magnetic resonance imaging MRI of the head is anticipated.[21] Finally, as with traditional sutures, the disadvantages of stapling include pain and the need to return for removal.

Hair Apposition Technique (HAT)

The HAT (also known as hair-ties) has the lowest cost and highest patient satisfaction for scalp repair.[1] Several strands of hair on either side of the wound are isolated, and a single *twist* of the hair is made (ie, no knot) and then secured with a drop of tissue adhesive, as illustrated in **Fig. 1**.[20] A video demonstrating the technique can be seen at https://lacerationrepair.com/alternative-wound-closure/hair-apposition-technique/.

For postrepair care, patients should avoid washing the wound for 2 days; the adhesive will then gradually flake off.[20] This technique should be used to repair linear, nonstellate lacerations of the scalp that are less than 10 cm in length. The patient must also have scalp hair greater than or equal to 3 cm in length. Hair-ties have a shorter procedure time, does not require shaving or removal of sutures or staples, and causes the patient minimal pain, leading to a higher patient acceptance rate for scalp lacerations compared with suturing.[20]

Secondary Intention

Healing by secondary intention is the oldest method for laceration repair or wound healing, but its use has declined since surgical techniques have been developed and refined. There is reluctance to use this method to its fullest advantage due to concerns for slow wound healing that could lead to pain, bleeding, infection, and scarring; however, wounds themselves are painless, and continued bleeding and new infection are rarely seen in wounds that are properly managed. Complications such as

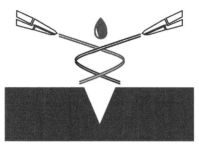

Fig. 1. Modified HAT, in which Kelly clamps are used to hold and twist the hair, rather than the clinician's fingers. (*Courtesy* of Michelle Lin, MD, Academic Life in Emergency Medicine, https://www.aliem.com/.)

hematomas, seromas, and suture reactions are also avoided.[23] Appropriate wounds that can close by secondary intention include wounds that have concern for infection (ie, closing such wounds would allow an infection to fester rather than drain) or wounds that are small, simple, superficial, and have good hemostasis.[21]. Wounds on concave surfaces (eg, nose, eye, ear, temple) result in a much better cosmetic result. A mature scar is hypopigmented and relatively avascular, making healed wounds less noticeable in light-colored skin than in darkly pigmented or telangiectatic skin. Older patients may also have better cosmetic result with secondary intention wound healing because of the laxity, irregular pigmentation, and wrinkles commonly found with their skin, allowing for scars to be better camouflaged.

Wound management requires an occlusive or semi-occlusive dressing with daily dressing changes that can be performed at home. A semi-occlusive environment keeps the wound clean and moist to prevent drying and crust formation, leading to improved reepithelization and minimizing pain. Patient counseling is recommended, though, as routine healing will cause mild redness, swelling, warmth, tenderness, and exudate surrounding the wound for a few millimeters. Concern for infection should be made if redness and swelling extend beyond a few millimeters from the wound or if there is purulent or foul-smelling drainage, fever, significant tenderness, or leukocytosis. Infection, though, is seen in less than 0.5% of wounds if kept properly occluded and cared for.[23]

OPERATIVE REPAIR
Contents of the Suture Kit

Whether purchased from a medical supply company or assembled from reusable materials, suture kits contain a needle driver (to hold the needle); pickups (forceps) with either serrated internal tips or hooks; small scissors; sterile gauze/sponges; and a small cup to hold tissue, used needles, or foreign bodies removed during wound exploration before closure. In addition, most commercially available kits also include a sterile 10 cc Luer lock syringe; an 18-gauge needle (for drawing up anesthetic); and a 25-, 27-, or 30-gauge needle (to inject the anesthetic).

Advantages and disadvantages of disposable and self-assembled kits

Commercially available disposable kits, while offering a low-cost solution (typically $5–10 per kit), often achieve this price point with lower-quality implements that are discarded after a single use. Consequently, many clinicians prefer reusable, stainless steel kits with higher-quality equipment that can be sterilized and allow for a smoother operative experience and can also be more cost-effective after multiple cycles of use.

Selection of Anesthetic

Choice of anesthetic depends on several factors, including wound location, depth, and the extent of the injury. The most common options in the primary care setting are lidocaine, bupivacaine, and LET (lidocaine-epinephrine-tetracaine) or EMLA (eutectic mixture of local anesthetics) creams. Select the anesthetic that balances cost, ease of administration, time needed (and available) for the procedure, and patient comfort.

Lidocaine

A variety of lidocaine preparations are available, including 1% with or without epinephrine and 2% viscous solution. Addition of epinephrine increases local vasoconstriction and increases duration of analgesia. It is an excellent choice for most areas of the body but some clinicians have been trained to avoid using epinephrine combinations in distal tissues—the tip of the nose, fingers, toes, and genitals—as these areas have restricted collateral blood flow and are more susceptible to ischemia with secondary necrosis. Although many investigators and lecturers have stated that no credible evidence backs up this theoretic complication, anecdotal reports abound and controversy persists. Viscous lidocaine can be used on mucosal surfaces but usually is less effective than LET or local infiltration.

Bupivacaine (Marcaine)

First discovered in 1957, bupivacaine is superior to lidocaine in analgesic effect and has a longer duration of action (4–6 hours vs 1–3 hours for lidocaine).[24,25] It is available in 0.25% and 0.5% concentrations and can be used in any area where lidocaine is an option.

LET and EMLA topical anesthetics

LET is an excellent topical anesthetic choice for superficial or moderately deep wounds. It is not contraindicated in open wounds and can be applied to wounds that have not yet been irrigated, making it appealing for use with fearful pediatric patients. If applied early, LET can decrease the length of stay. The onset of effect is 15 to 30 minutes and LET costs approximately $1 to 2 per application.

By comparison, EMLA has a slower onset of action (up to 1 hour) and is more expensive ($8–16 per application). Topical application of EMLA cream may be associated with rare instances of methemoglobinemia.

Use of a topical anesthetic may allow for the elimination of (or at least a reduced need for) injected anesthetic. Decreased use of supplies (ie, syringes, needles, sharps containers), decreased pain for the patient, and higher patient and clinician satisfaction result. However, the onset of action is much slower than either lidocaine or bupivacaine injections, which may be impractical in a busy facility.

Anesthesia Techniques

Before injection of anesthetic, ensure that the wound has been modestly irrigated to prevent secondary contamination. Warming lidocaine or bupivacaine to room temperature can reduce patient discomfort when instilling the anesthetic.[26] Some practices use lidocaine buffered with sodium bicarbonate for the same reason.[27] Use the finest (smallest) gauge needle possible (ie, 27 or 30 gauge): Needles larger than 25-gauge can increase tissue distension and pain for the patient. Allow at least 15 minutes for the anesthetic to take effect, although typically satisfactory anodynia is achieved within 5 minutes.[28]

Three basic anesthesia techniques are detailed here: local infiltration, field, and digital blocks. More advanced techniques include tendon sheath and facial nerve blocks; further information of these approaches can be found at the New York School of Regional Anesthesia (https://www.nysora.com).

Local infiltration
This foundational technique involves administration of anesthetic into the edges of the wound, just beneath the epidermis (and deeper layers, if necessary).

Field blocks
Often used for contaminated wounds, skin abscesses, and where tissue distortion would otherwise make tissue repair difficult (eg, the vermillion border), this technique attempts to numb a diamond-shaped region of tissue using 1 or 2 injections.

Digital block
Injuries to the fingers and toes are quite common; targeting the lateral and medial aspects of the nerve branches at the base of the digit can provide anesthesia without distorting the tissue in need of repair. Because the injection itself is proximal to the wound, be sure to clean the unbroken skin at the injection site with an alcohol swab. Variations to this approach include also injecting the dorsal aspects with or without the palmar side. Take care not to inject the digital artery.

Selection of Suture Material

Suture material comes in a variety of gauges and lengths and with different shapes and types of connected needles. In general clinic practice, the fiber diameter will typically range between 0.1 and 0.3 mm, corresponding to 6 to 0 and 3 to 0 designations by the United States Pharmacopeia (USP). Finer material, commonly used in ophthalmologic applications, can use 10 to 0 USP (0.02 mm); thicker threads for obstetric or orthopedic procedures go from 0 to 4 USP (without the "-0" suffix) or higher. Selection of suture gauge is a balance between sufficient tensile strength (for the best recovery of function) and the finest material possible (for the best cosmetic outcome).

Suture thread itself is either nonabsorbable or absorbable, and selection depends on the nature of the wound itself, as well as the patient (eg, what is their preference, are they likely to return as requested, can they appropriately care for the wound).

Nonabsorbable material—nylon (brand-name Ethilon) or polyethylene (brand-name Prolene)—is typically the suture of choice for superficial closure in patients able to follow-up reliably. The thread is easy to handle, generally does not cause inflammation, and has very good tensile strength. Prolene, which is typically blue in color, may be preferable in hair-bearing areas, as it is more easily distinguished from the patient's own hair. Silk, which is also nonabsorbable, is rarely used due to subsequent inflammatory reaction to the foreign protein.

Absorbable sutures, as listed in **Box 2**, should be considered in deeper layers of repair, pediatric patients, and other patients for whom follow-up for suture removal may pose significant challenge. Synthetic absorbable sutures are usually made from polyglycolic acid; gut sutures are literally made from cow or sheep intestine.

Preparing the Surgical Field

After cleaning the wound and applying local anesthesia, don appropriate gloves and isolate the affected body part, placing an absorbent pad beneath and using a fenestrated (window) sterile drape. The patient should be advised not to touch the drapes unless told to, and both the patient and the clinician should be positioned in such a way that is comfortable for both parties for a prolonged period. Recent research has suggested the operator's gloves need not be sterile.[29,30] A preprocedure check

| Box 2 |
| Absorbable suture thread and its best use |
| Polyglactin 910 (brand-name Vicryl)—fascia, muscle, or deep tissue layers |
| Chromic gut—mucosal surfaces (eg, inner lip and mouth) |
| Brand-name Vicryl Rapide—superficial wounds (particularly facial lacerations) |
| Fast-absorbing gut—superficial wounds (particularly facial lacerations) |

list can be used to improve efficiency and reduce errors. Good lighting is important, and clinicians may consider using store-bought reading glasses as a proxy for surgical loupes when fine, close repair in areas of high cosmetic consequence (eg, the face) is needed.

Approach to Wound Closure

There is an adage in suture repair: approximate, do not strangulate. The goal of operative laceration repair is to bring together the edges of the wound to facilitate healing, not to tighten the sutures to the point that they cause tissue ischemia. The clinician should use their equipment in a way that is both comfortable and safe. Use a needle-driver to hold the needle just after the connection point to the thread and forceps to evert the skin edges; using one's fingers directly can result in needle-stick injuries. The clinician should have good support for their upper extremities and strive to make all movements using only the wrists and fingers; this will result in greater accuracy and reduced fatigue.

The needle generally enters the tissue surface at a 90° angle. Whenever possible, the repair should begin in the middle of the wound, bisecting the laceration length with each subsequent suture, as shown in **Fig. 2**; this allows more even distribution of tension and avoids malalignment (known in some circles as a "dog ear") that results in poor cosmesis. The distance between sutures—as well as the overall number of sutures—depends most on the tension of the site. Multilevel repairs should use thicker (resorbable) suture in the deeper layers; this is where the lion's share of tension reduction is accomplished. In general, the number of knots (throws) for each suture is the same or one more than the suture caliber. For instance, 4-0 suture would be tied off with a minimum of 4 or 5 knots.

The number of sutures placed in each layer should be documented to facilitate removal later. (Typically, the patient wants to know as well.) Retained nonabsorbable sutures can result in granulomatous changes, poor cosmesis, and/or infection.

Suture Techniques

The 3 most common operative wound closure techniques are illustrated in **Fig. 3**.

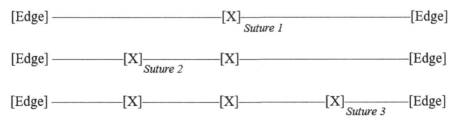

Fig. 2. Sutures should be placed halfway between the wound edge and previous stitch.

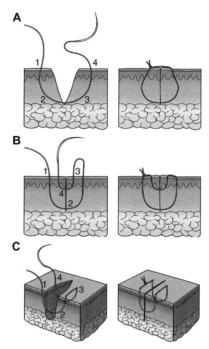

Fig. 3. Operative wound closure techniques. (*A*) Simple interrupted. (*B*) Vertical mattress. (*C*) Horizontal mattress. (*Modified from* Percy A. Chapter 4: Procedures. In: Kleinman K, McDaniel L, Molly M, eds. Harriet Lane Handbook. 22nd ed. Elsevier; 2021:61-97.)

Simple interrupted closure

This technique is easy to master, excellent for approximating even moderately tense wounds, and can be applied to almost every wound encountered in clinic. It can be slower to use than running or running-locking techniques (not covered in this article), especially with larger wounds. The suture thread enters and exits the skin only once per stitch.

Horizontal mattress closure

With suture thread running parallel to the wound, the interrupted horizontal mattress suture is ideal for gaping or high-tension wounds. It can be used in both superficial and deep layers and is particularly useful for reapproximating lacerated muscle or fascial layers. It is also a helpful technique to use with fragile skin, especially where simple interrupted sutures would tend to "pull through" the skin. As the interrupted vertical mattress suture, this closure provides excellent wound margin eversion with improved cosmesis compared with the simple interrupted technique.

Vertical mattress closure

As with the interrupted vertical mattress suture is used in body sites where the wound edges tend to invert, for example, wounds on concave surfaces (eg, posterior neck). It helps reduce tension on the suture thread and may yield improved cosmetic outcomes. It does tend to be slower to perform than simple interrupted closure, however.

The suture needle enters and exits the tissue 4 times, perpendicular to the wound, using the "far-far-near-near" system: the "far" entry starts approximately 4 to 8 mm from the wound margin and is inserted fairly deep into the dermis. The needle is then passed through the other side and out of the tissue, the same distance on the opposite side of the initial placement. The needle is then grasped with the needle driver in the reverse orientation, entering "near" in the same vertical plane and passing through and back out the other side of the wound once more, where it is tied.

Wound Dressing

Once the wound repair is complete, the area should be gently cleansed of topical anti-microbial solution, blood, and other debris using a damp gauze pad. If nonabsorbable sutures were used, topical antibiotic ointment should be applied, followed by a non-adherent dressing (eg, brand-name Telfa pad) and a cling/elastic dressing (eg, brand-name Coban) to keep it in place (as well as prevent the wound from being disturbed by a curious patient). Twenty-four hours after the repair, the patient can gently wash the area with soap and water. They should avoid submerging the wound, however, as this can wrinkle the skin and ruin the repair. The patient should be encouraged to reapply antibiotic ointment (or petroleum jelly) and change the wound dressing daily or when visibly soiled.[31]

SCAR-MINIMIZING TECHNIQUES

A scar is an exuberant healing response resulting from overgrowth of fibrous tissue when skin has been damaged. The risk of a thickened scar is higher in certain high-pressure body sites such as the shoulder, scapula, anterior chest, lower abdomen, earlobe, and any area overlying a bony prominence. Patients of Afro-Caribbean descent and those with personal or family history of scarring are also at high risk for excessive scarring.[32] Three main treatment methods are thought to have a beneficial influence on the cosmetic outcome of scars: wound support, hydration, and hastened maturity of scars. Therefore, to minimize scar formation, systemic conditions should be optimized, and minimal trauma or inflammation should be caused during the repair and healing of the wound.[32,33] A mature scar is hypopigmented, so it is important for patients to avoid excessive sunlight exposure to prevent sunburning or increased inflammation of the scar site. Several therapies have been discussed to help minimize scarring and improve the cosmetic appearance of a healed wound including scar massage, vitamin E, onion extract preparations, adhesive tape support, and corticosteroids; however, a sufficiently evidence-based method has not been identified at this time.[32]

Scar Massage

Scar massage increases scar pliability and decreases scar banding leading to improved skin quality, relieved sensitivity, increased cutaneous hydration, and better acceptance of the lesion. Scar massage is contraindicated in fragile skin or wounds that are open, infected, painful, or have significant inflammation.[33]

Vitamin E

Vitamin E applied topically penetrates the dermis and subcutaneous tissue and is believed to improve cosmetic outcome of scars via antioxidant properties.[32,33] Topical vitamin E, though, may worsen scars by causing contact urticaria, eczematous dermatitis, erythema multiforme-like reactions, and contact dermatitis. Because of the mixed evidence, there is little scientific support for vitamin E in the literature.[33] Anecdotal reports suggest using vitamin E lotion for 6 months may reduce ultraviolet-induced scarring and hyperpigmentation.

Onion Extract Preparations

Onion extract preparations (eg, brand-name Mederma cream) may accelerate wound healing by exerting effects on mast cells and fibroblasts in the inflammatory cascade to decrease inflammation.[32] The bioflavonoid component from the onion extract further has antiproliferative effects through antihistamine properties; this normalizes or decreases collagen production by fibroblasts leading to reduced dermal scar volume and relative normalization of the scar maturation process leading to less inflammation, erythema, and scar hypertrophy.[34] A recent study, though, comparing Mederma with a petroleum-based emollient (eg, brand-name Aquaphor ointment) did not improve scar cosmesis or symptomatology.[33]

Adhesive Tape Support

Wounds are susceptible to skin tension after suture (or equivalent) removal. Nonstretch, microporous, hypoallergenic paper tape may then be used after 2 weeks to control scar tension through eliminating stretching forces to prevent hypertrophic scarring. Tape with an elastic component may be useful for scars over mobile or complex surfaces such as joints. For benefit, tape may need to be used for several weeks. Notably, tape may cause a localized red rash due to adhesives; however, these reactions are often minor and typically resolve spontaneously.[33]

Corticosteroids

Corticosteroids suppress inflammation by inhibiting fibroblast proliferation that leads to collagen synthesis, causing vasoconstriction that limits wound oxygenation and nutrition, transforming growth factors and collagen in keratinocytes, and promoting collagen degeneration. Intralesional steroid therapy often has adverse effects including dermal atrophy and hypopigmentation, making intralesional triamcinolone first-line treatment only for treatment of hypertrophic and keloid scars. Topical corticosteroids have failed to reduce scar tissue formation and are not advocated due to lack of evidence-based literature.[32]

FOLLOW-UP CARE

When instructing a patient where and when to return for a wound check and/or removal of staples or nonabsorbable sutures, several factors should be considered: wound location (eg, high-tension repairs over joints), the patient's age, and other elements that would predict poor healing (eg, underlying metabolic disease, chronic use of immunosuppressants, poor perfusion, alcohol or substance abuse). Clinical judgment usually outweighs textbook estimates.

Signs and Symptoms of Infection

Patients should be counseled on the signs and symptoms of wound infection (eg, erythema, edema, warmth, worsening pain, spread of these signs beyond the immediate laceration repair site) and that they serve as reasons to seek reevaluation. Some patients misinterpret granulation tissue (or allergic reaction to triple antibiotic ointment) as a sign of infection. Purulent drainage and discharge, especially in the presence of systemic symptoms such as fevers and rigors, should also be evaluated urgently. Wounds at high risk for infection (eg, contaminated wounds, bite wounds, patients with immunocompromise or diabetes mellitus) should be followed-up closely, ideally with scheduled follow-up within the first 48 to 72 hours after injury.

Table 1	
Timing for suture removal based on body location	
Location	Timing of Suture Removal
Face	3–5 days
Eyelids	5 days (3 days for low-tension, up to 7 days for high-tension)
Neck	5 days
Scalp	7–10 days
Arms	7–14 days
Trunk	7–14 days
Legs	8–10 days
Digits, palms, or soles	10–14 days

Data from Refs [1,21,35,36]

Suture Removal

Lacerations repaired with absorbable suture do not necessarily need to have follow-up if uncomplicated and the suture material is absorbed appropriately. The timing of nonabsorbable suture and staple removal depends on the location and site of laceration repair, as seen in **Table 1**. These recommendations are based on expert opinion and personal experience with laceration repairs.

In general, a pair of forceps and either suture scissors or a #11 blade scalpel (with the sharp edge pointing upwards) are the only pieces of equipment needed to remove sutures. A single cut in the loop portion of the suture should be made to avoid leaving foreign material embedded.

Staple Removal

It is important to make sure the clinician removing staples has the appropriate staple remover device. The anticipated interval between application and removal of staples is very similar to those listed above.[36]

To remove staples, make sure the remover is positioned with both prongs under the staple. Next, depress the handle in order to bend the staple outward in the midline. Carefully ease the staple out of the skin and clean any drainage and/or bleeding.[36]

Tissue Adhesive Removal

Patients whose wounds were repaired using tissue adhesive typically do not need to follow-up for adhesive removal. Cyanoacrylates typically will peel off within 5 to 10 days, once the epithelial layer sloughs off. If the adhesive does not peel off on its own, petroleum jelly or antibiotic ointment can be applied to facilitate removal.[37] As with other methods of wound closure, patients who had tissue adhesive wound closure and express concern for infection or inappropriate healing should seek reevaluation.[37]

PEARLS AND PITFALLS (CLINICS CARE POINTS)

1. Despite being used in common practice, sterile normal saline is no more efficacious than tap water for wound irrigation and avoidance of infection.[5]

2. Similarly, sterile gloves have not been shown to afford lower infection rates with repair of uncomplicated lacerations, compared to nonsterile gloves.[30]

3. Foreign bodies composed of plastic or wood may be missed on plain radiographs, whereas glass, metal (except aluminum), and stone should be visualized. When in doubt, an ultrasound may be helpful.[38,39]

4. Debate exists over whether animal bite wounds should be treated with prophylactic antibiotics and, separately, permitted to close by secondary intention. Wounds at higher risk for infection (eg, on the hand) probably warrant both of these approaches.[40]

5. Although tissue adhesives used in medical clinics generally do not "sting" when applied to a wound, polymerization is an exothermic reaction, which can be frightening to young children.[41,42]

6. When applying staples, be certain to have a staple remover available both at the time of the initial closure but again for later removal.

7. Reluctance to use lidocaine with epinephrine for local anesthesia in distal tissues may be based on historic concern (with procaine). That said, injected phentolamine can be used to reverse ischemia if it were to occur.[43-46]

8. Positioning of the patient undergoing laceration repair should be comfortable for both them and the clinician. The operative field should be well-lit, and inexpensive magnifying tools can be used for better visualization in delicate areas.

DEDICATION

This article is dedicated in the memory of Beth Marie Tallman (née Nass), FNP (1987–2021).

DISCLOSURE

The authors have nothing to disclose. Dr K. Bernstein is current, active duty of the United States Navy. The views expressed in this article are those of the authors and do not necessarily reflect the official policy or position of the Department of the Navy, Department of Defense, or the United States Government.

REFERENCES

1. Forsch RT, Little SH, Williams C. Laceration repair: a practical approach. Am Fam Physician 2017;95(10):628–36.
2. Moscati RM, Mayrose J, Reardon RF, et al. A multicenter comparison of tap water versus sterile saline for wound irrigation. Acad Emerg Med 2007;14(5):404–9.
3. Nordt S, Swadron S. Your [sic] going to irrigate that wound with what?? *Urgent Care RAP* (podcast). 2015. Available at: https://www.hippoed.com/urgentcare/rap/episode/yourgoingto/journalclub. Accessed September 1, 2021.
4. Valente JH, Forti RJ, Freundlich LF, et al. Wound irrigation in children: saline solution or tape water? Ann Emerg Med 2003;41(5):609–16.
5. Weiss EA, Oldham G, Lin M, et al. Water is a safe and effective alternative to sterile normal saline for wound irrigation prior to suturing: a prospective, double-blind, randomized, controlled clinical trial. BMJ Open 2013;3(1):e001504.
6. Ernst AA, Gershoff L, Miller P. Warmed versus room temperature saline for laceration irrigation: a randomized clinical trial. South Med J 2003;96(5):436–9.
7. Nicks BA, Ayello EA, Woo K, et al. Acute wound management: revisiting the approach to assessment, irrigation, and closure considerations. Int J Emerg Med 2010;3(4):399–407.

8. Tsao S. Basic wound management. CDEM curriculum. Available at: https://www.saem.org/about-saem/academies-interest-groups-affiliates2/cdem/for-students/online-education/m3-curriculum/group-emergency-department-procedures/basic-wound-management Page. Accessed September 1, 2021.

9. Tandberg D. Glass in the hand and foot. Will an X-ray film show it? JAMA 1982; 248(15):1872–4.

10. No author. Tetanus. Available at: https://www.cdc.gov/tetanus/clinicians.html Page. Accessed May 30, 2021.

11. Havers FP, Moro PL, Hunter P, et al. Use of tetanus toxoid, reduced diphtheria toxoid, and acellular pertussis vaccines: updated recommendations of the Advisory Committee on Immunization Practices – United States, 2019. MMWR Morb Mortal Weekly Rep 2020;67:77.

12. Liang JL, Tiwari T, Moro P, et al. Prevention of pertussis, tetanus, and diphtheria with vaccines in the United States: recommendations of the Advisory Committee on Immunization Practices (ACIP). MMWR Recomm Rep 2018;67:1.

13. Waterbook AL, Hiller K, Hays DP, et al. Do topical antibiotics help prevent infection in minor traumatic uncomplicated soft tissue wounds? Ann Emerg Med 2013;61:86.

14. Wieczorkiewicz SM, Sincak CA, editors. The Pharmacist's guide to antimicrobial therapy and Stewardship. Bethesda: ASHP; 2016.

15. Diaz JH. Skin and soft tissue infections following marine injuries and exposures in travelers. J Trav Med 2014;21:207.

16. Noonburg GE. Management of extremity trauma and related infections occurring in the aquatic environment. J Am Acad Orthop Surg 2005;13:243.

17. Jaindl M, Grünauer J, Platzer P, et al. The management of bite wounds in children – a retrospective analysis at a level I trauma centre. Injury 2013;43:2117.

18. Paschos NK, Makris EA, Gantsos A, et al. Primary closure versus non-closure of dog bite wounds, a randomized controlled trial. Injury 2014;45(1):237–40.

19. Rui-feng C, Li-song H, Ji-bo Z, et al. Emergency treatment on facial laceration of dog bite wounds with immediate primary closure: a prospective randomized trial study. BMC Emerg Med 2013;13(Supple 1):S2.

20. Hock M, Ooi S, Saw S, et al. A randomized controlled trial comparing the hair apposition technique with tissue glue to standard suturing in scalp lacerations (HAT study). Ann Emerg Med 2002;40(1):19–26.

21. Forsch R. Essentials of skin laceration repair. Am Fam Physician 2008;78(8): 945–52.

22. Singer AJ, Quinn JV, Clark RE, et al. Closure of lacerations and incisions with octylcyanoacrylate: a multicenter randomized controlled trial. Surgery 2002;131(3):270–6.

23. Zitelli J. Secondary intention healing: an alternative to surgical repair. Clin Derm 1984;2(3):92–106.

24. Moradi S, Naghavi N. Comparison of bupivacaine and lidocaine use for postoperative pain control in endodontics. Iran Endod J 2010;5(1):31–5.

25. Velioglu O, Calis AS, Koca H, et al. Bupivacaine vs lidocaine: a comparison of local anesthetic efficacy in impacted third molar surgery. Clin Oral Invest 2020; 24:3539–46.

26. Jones JS, Plzak C, Wynn BN, et al. Effective of temperature and pH adjustment of bupivacaine for intradermal anesthesia. Am J Emerg Med 1998;16(2):117–20.

27. Vent A, Surber C, Graf Johansen NT, et al. Buffered lidocaine 1%/epinephrine 1:100,000 with sodium bicarbonate (sodium hydrogen carbonate) in a 3:1 ratio is less painful than a 9:1 ratio: a double-blind, randomized, placebo-controlled, crossover trial. J Am Acad Dermatol 2020;83(1):159–65.

28. Latham JL, Martin SN. Infiltrative anesthesia in office practice. Am Fam Physician 2014;89(12):956–62.
29. Brewer JD, Gonzalez AB, Baum CL, et al. Comparison of sterile vs nonsterile gloves in cutaneous surgery and common outpatient dental procedures: a systematic review and meta-analysis. JAMA Dermatol 2016;152(9):1008–14.
30. Perelman VS, Francis GJ, Rutledge T, et al. Sterile versus nonsterile gloves for repair of uncomplicated lacerations in the emergency department: a randomized controlled trial. Ann Emerg Med 2004;43(3):362–70.
31. Smack DP, Harrington AC, Dunn C, et al. Infection and allergy incidence in ambulatory surgery patients using white petrolatum vs bacitracin ointment, a randomized controlled trial. JAMA 1996;276(12):972–7.
32. Tziotzios C, Profyris C, Sterling J. Cutaneous scarring: pathophysiology, molecular mechanisms, and scar reduction therapeutics – part II, strategies to reduce scar formation after dermatologic procedures. J Am Acad Derm 2012;66(1): 13–24.
33. Atiyeh B. Nonsurgical management of hypertrophic scars: evidence-based therapies, standard practices, and emergency methods. Aesth Plast Surg 2007;31: 468–92.
34. Sidgwick GP, McGeorge D, Bayat A. A comprehensive evidence-based review on the role of topicals and dressings in the management of skin scarring. Arch Derm Res 2015;307(6):461–77.
35. Lamers RL, Scrimshaw LE. Methods of wound closure. In: Roberts JR, Custalow CB, Thomsen TW, editors. Clinical procedures in Emergency medicine. 7th ed. Philadelphia: Elsevier; 2019. p. 655.
36. McNamara R, DeAngelis M. Laceration repair with sutures, staples, and wound closure tapes. In: King C, Henretig FM, editors. Textbook of pediatric Emergency procedures, 1005, 2nd edition. Philadelphia: Lippincott Williams & Wilkins; 2008. p. 1034.
37. Bruns TB, Worthington JM. Using tissue adhesive for wound repair: a practical guide to Dermabond. Am Fam Physician 2000;61:1383.
38. Hunter TB, Taljanovic MS. Foreign bodies. RadioGraphics 2003;23(3):731–57.
39. Voss JO, Maier C, Wüster J, et al. Imaging foreign bodies in head and neck trauma: a pictorial review. Insights Imaging 2021;12(1):20.
40. Ellis R, Ellis C. Dog and cat bites. Am Fam Physician 2014;90(4):239–43.
41. Tissue adhesive for the topical approximation of skin – class II special controls guidance for industry and FDA staff. 2008. Available at: https://www.fda.gov/medical-devices/guidance-documents-medical-devices-and-radiation-emitting-products/tissue-adhesive-topical-approximation-skin-class-ii-special-controls-guidance-industry-and-fda-staff. Accessed June 21, 2021.
42. Rivera RF, Fagan M. Laceration repair. In: Olympia R, O'Neill R, Silvis M, editors. Urgent Care Medicine Secrets. 1st edition. Philadelphia: Elsevier; 2018. ch.44.
43. Denkler K. A comprehensive review of epinephrine in the finger: To do or not to do. Plast Reconstr Surg 2001;108(1):114–24.
44. Denkler K. Myth of not using lidocaine with epinephrine in the digits. Am Fam Physician 2008;81(10):1188.
45. Ruiter T, Harter T, Miladore N, et al. Finger amputation after injection with lidocaine and epinephrine. Eplasty 2014;14:ic43.
46. Thomson CJ, Lalonde DH, Denkler KA, et al. A critical look at the evidence for and against elective epinephrine use in the finger. Plast Reconstr Surg 2007; 119(1):260–6.

Abscess Incision and Drainage

Jaime K. Bowman, MD, FAAFP

KEYWORDS

- Tissue abscess • Incision and drainage • Perianal abscess • Hidradenitis

KEY POINTS

- Simple abscesses may be safely managed by primary care physicians in the office through incision and drainage.
- Wound culture and antibiotics are rarely indicated. Wound packing may improve healing of larger abscesses.
- Refer oral, perianal, and abscesses associated with hidradenitis suppurativa.

INTRODUCTION AND PATHOPHYSIOLOGY

An abscess is a localized collection of purulent material surrounded by inflammation and granulation in response to an infectious source, typically *Staphylococcus aureus* or streptococcal species.[1] Furuncles or boils are abscesses formed at the site of a sweat gland or hair follicle. The most common sites for abscess formation are in areas of skin friction or minor trauma (extremities, buttocks, breast, axilla, groin) that allow for disruption of the protective skin barrier and entry for microorganisms. Risk factors include older age, cardiopulmonary or hepatorenal disease, diabetes mellitus, debility, immunosenescence or immunocompromise, obesity, peripheral arteriovenous or lymphatic insufficiency, and trauma. Cellulitis, skin necrosis, sinus tracks, and scarring can occur with abscess formation. In some locations, such as the perianal region, gram-negative, anaerobic, and enteric organisms can contribute.

A small abscess (<5 mm or 0.2 in) or one within 4 mm (0.15 in) of the skin surface may resolve with warm compresses or antibiotics or may drain spontaneously. When an abscess enlarges, the collection of pus and inflammation can increase tissue tension limiting blood flow and reducing the efficacy of conservative treatments. Incision and drainage (I & D) is indicated to remove the infection and inflammation, relieve the pressure, and resolve the pathologic condition. Postprocedure trimethoprim/sulfamethoxazole (TMP-SMX) decreases the risk of treatment failure and recurrence

Department of Medical Education and Clinical Sciences, Washington State University, 412 East Spokane Falls Boulevard, Spokane, WA 99202-1495, USA
E-mail address: Jaime.bowman@wsu.edu

Prim Care Clin Office Pract 49 (2022) 39–45
https://doi.org/10.1016/j.pop.2021.10.002
0095-4543/22/© 2021 Elsevier Inc. All rights reserved.

with fewer side effects than clindamycin.[2] Special cases for consideration are discussed specifically.

PRESENTATION AND DIAGNOSIS

The diagnosis of an abscess is made upon clinical examination. Patients typically present with erythema, warmth, edema, and pain over the site. Abscesses will frequently have a concentrated nodule of fluctuance sometimes with central blanching.

Point-of-care ultrasonography (POCUS) may help differentiate between cellulitis infections and soft tissue abscesses when clinical examination is not clear. POCUS measures the abscess and how deep it lies under the surface of the skin, guiding the choice to proceed with I & D (or treating conservatively with oral antibiotics and hot compresses). POCUS also helps guide the planning of the incision and the assessment of the adequacy of drainage, leading to fewer procedure failures.[3]

Rarely, patients will present with systemic features of infection including fever, tachycardia, diaphoresis, fatigue, anorexia, nausea, and vomiting. These features are more common in immunocompromised patients and may warrant evaluation with blood cultures, tissue culture, complete blood cell count, C-reactive protein level, and liver and kidney function tests.[1]

REFERRAL CONSIDERATIONS

Most simple abscesses can safely be managed in the ambulatory office with the exception of those that involve the face, hands, or genitalia. In these cases, consultation and hospitalization may be advantageous.[1] Extensively large, deep, or necrotic abscesses may require surgical debridement and general anesthesia.[4] Patients with compromised immunity may require close observation and tissue culture.[5]

INFORMED CONSENT

Informed consent should include the following:

1. Description of the procedure: incision of the skin to allow drainage of the infection.
2. Indications: drainage of skin infection.
3. Risks: bleeding, worsening infection, pain, scarring, need for further surgical intervention, incomplete treatment, and persistence of infection.
4. Benefits: confirming diagnosis, treating infection, and relieving pain.
5. Alternatives: trial of medication and observation.
6. Prognosis without treatment: rarely do abscesses resolve without intervention, occasionally they will rupture, but most often they worsen or spread.
7. Patient rights: time to make decision, ability to obtain second opinion, and to refuse recommended treatment.

EQUIPMENT

- Gloves (nonsterile), 2 pairs per provider
- Gown
- Eye protection or splash guard
- Povidone-iodine or chlorhexidine solution
- Sterile drape
- Local anesthetic (1% to 2% lidocaine with or without epinephrine)
- Syringe with 12- to 14-gauge needle (to draw anesthetic) and 25- to 30 gauge needle (for injection)

- 4 × 4-in gauze
- No. 11 or 15 blade or 4-mm punch biopsy
- Curved hemostats
- Curet
- Dressing of choice

If wound requires packing, add:

- Iodoform gauze (3/8–1 inch width)
- Bandage scissors

SITE PREPARATION, STERILE TECHNIQUE

1. Provider should don proper personal protective equipment, including gloves, gown, and eye protection or facial splash guard. The use of sterile gloves does not change the outcome of the procedure.[6]
2. The surface of the abscess and surrounding skin should be cleansed with povidone-iodine or chlorhexidine solution.
3. Sterile draping should be used if indicated.
4. Gloves should be changed before initiating field block.

ANESTHESIA

Perform a field block with 1% to 2% lidocaine without epinephrine. Epinephrine is not indicated because the tissue pressure supports hemostasis. Traditional teaching has held that epinephrine is contraindicated in tissues with one arterial source (eg, fingers, toes, ears, penis, nose), although the evidence does not necessarily support this practice.[7] Assure injection into tissues alongside and below the abscess (**Fig. 1**) avoiding instilling liquid into the cavity of abscess or it may rupture the wall or tissue planes due to excessive pressure. Abscesses are acidic and anesthesia can lose effectiveness more quickly.

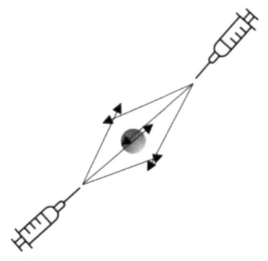

Fig. 1. Field block anesthesia.

TECHNIQUE

Once the patient has fully consented, the site is cleansed, the provider has donned appropriate personal protective equipment, and anesthesia (field block) is adequate, proceed with I & D.

1. At point of maximal fluctuance, create an incision deep and long enough to allow cavity to drain (typically, at least 4 mm wide and through cavity wall) with either a punch biopsy (**Fig. 2**) or a No. 11 or 15 blade scalpel (**Fig. 3**). Punch biopsies can reduce the size of the incision while more adequately allowing drainage and reducing early closure. When able, following the lines of Langerhans lessens tension and scaring.
2. Allow purulent contents to drain. Explore the abscess cavity with sterile swab and/or curved hemostats to break up loculations, explore any fistulas, and ensure no foreign bodies. To avoid potential injury due to retained sharp foreign body, do not use gloved finger. Culturing of the contents is not routinely indicated. Irrigation of the cavity is also not indicated.[8]
3. When the abscess is greater than 5 cm (1.97 inches) in diameter, packing may be indicated to allow escape of inflammation while healing and closure of wound by secondary intention. Abscesses less than 5 cm do not require packing.[9] Grasp packing with curved hemostat and feed packing into the cavity, filling it from the back to the incision (**Fig. 4**). Leave 1 to 2 cm (0.5 in) outside of the wound for ease of removal and wicking of purulent fluid.
4. Cover with a clean, dry dressing such as 4 × 4-inch gauze. Do not occlude.
5. Follow-up packed wounds every 24 to 48 hours to change dressing, remove packing, and assess for repacking. Large absences may require repacking several times to heal fully. Wounds without packing may not require follow-up if simple and small.

HEMOSTASIS

In all but rare cases, bleeding will be minimal. Profuse bleeding may complicate when venous or artery structures are damaged.

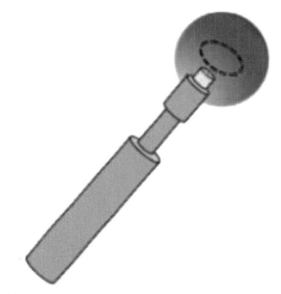

Fig. 2. Punch incision.

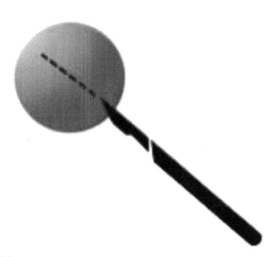

Fig. 3. Scalpel incision.

CLOSURE

Incisions after abscess drainage are left open to heal by secondary intention. Scarring is common. Clinical trials are underway that suggest primary closure may result in faster healing times without increased recurrence, and further evidence is needed to change current practice guidelines.[10]

SPECIAL CASES
Oral Abscesses

Oral abscesses frequently result from underlying dental carries. As tooth decay progresses, it infects the dental pulp, which communicates with surrounding soft tissue. Management of oral abscesses frequently requires incision, drainage, tooth extraction, and/or root canal as well as antibiotic treatment; this should be managed with a dental professional. In severe cases, progressing infections can involve the facial planes of the face and neck and become a medical emergency, especially if the airway becomes compromised.[11]

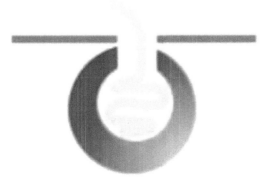

Fig. 4. Wound packing.

Perianal Abscesses

Perianal abscesses are associated with inflammatory bowel disease and HIV and are frequently an idiopathic infection of the cryptoglobular glands. Perianal abscesses have high rates of complications, most notably perianal fistula formation. Standard of care includes early and urgent referral for surgical drainage, exploration under anesthesia, and avoiding empirical antibiotic use.[12]

Hidradenitis Suppurativa

The abscesses associated with hidradenitis suppurativa (HS) almost always have complex sinus formation and relapse frequently.[13] When abscesses form in deep skin folds with hair and apocrine glands, such as the axilla, perineum, perianal, buttocks, scrotum, and submammary areas, consider HS. Multiple nodules are commonly present. HS is a severe dermatologic condition of inflammatory spreading through the subcutaneous tissue planes, superinfection, and chronic painful, odiferous draining sinus tracks with fibrosis and scarring. A multidisciplinary approach including a primary care clinician and specialist is recommended.[13]

COMPLICATIONS

- Recurrence of abscess is common (up to 19% of patients)[14]
- Scarring
- Inadequate anesthesia
- Pain during and after the procedure
- Bleeding
- Septic thromboembolism
- Necrotizing fasciitis
- Fistula formation
- Damage to nerves and blood vessels

FOLLOW-UP

With wound packing: every 24 to 48 hours to change dressing and assess need for repacking unless able to perform packing and dressing changes at home.

Without wound packing: as needed depending on the size of abscess and comorbid conditions.

Postprocedure TMP-SMX decreases the risk of treatment failure and recurrence with fewer side effects than clindamycin.[2]

CLINICS CARE POINTS

- Frequent or complex abscess formation may indicate immunity compromise
- Culturing the contents of a simple abscess is not routinely recommended
- Systemic features of infection may warrant sepsis evaluation and hospitalization
- Referral is needed when abscesses occur in the mouth or perianal area and when associated with HS
- Packing the cavity of abscesses less than 5 cm (1.97 in) does not prevent further need for I & D
- Abscess wounds should not be closed; they should be allowed to heal by secondary intention

DISCLOSURE

The author has nothing to disclose.

REFERENCES

1. Kalyanakrishnan Ramakrishnan M, ROBERT C, SALINAS M, NELSON IVAN AGU-DELO HIGUITA M. Skin and soft tissue infections. Am Fam Physician 2015;92(6): 474–83.
2. Vermandere M, Aertgeerts B, Agoritsas T. Antibiotics after incision and drainage for uncomplicated skin abscesses: a clinical practice guideline. BMJ 2018;360.
3. Romolo J Gaspari AS. Abscess incision and drainage with or without ultrasonography: a randomized controlled trial. Ann Emerg Med 2019;1–7.
4. Heidi Wimberly, P.-C. (2021). Incision and Drainage of Abscesses. 5 Minute Consult.
5. Daniel J, Derkson M. Incision and drainage of an abscess. In: John GC, Pfenninger L, editors. Procedures for primary care physicians. St. Louis: Mosby; 1994. p. 50–3.
6. Jerry D Brewer AB. Comparison of sterile vs nonsterile gloves in cutaneous surgery and common outpatient dental procedures: a systematic review and meta-analysis. J Am Med Assoc - Dermatol 2016;152(9):1008–14.
7. Hans-Martin Häfner MR. Epinephrine-supplemented local anesthetics for ear and nose surgery: clinical use without complications in more than 10,000 surgical procedures. J German Soc Dermatol 2005;3(3):195–9.
8. Hendey BC. Irrigation of cutaneous abscesses does not improve treatment success. Ann Emerg Med 2016;67(3):379–83.
9. O'Bright NE. Packing versus non-packing outcomes for abscesses after incision and drainage. J Okla State Med Assoc 2017;110(2):78–9.
10. Singer AJ. Primary closure of cutaneous abscesses: a systematic review. Am J Emerg Med 2011;29(4):361–6.
11. Stephens MB, Wiedemer JP, Kushner GM. Dental problems in primary care. Am Fam Physician 2018;98(11):54–660.
12. Sahnan K, Adegbola SO, Tozer PJ, et al. Perianal abscess. BMJ 2017 Feb 21; 356:j475. https://doi.org/10.1136/bmj.j475.
13. Alikhan Me. North American clinical management guidelines for hidradenitis suppurativa: a publication from the United States and Canadian Hidradenitis Suppurativa Foundations. J Am Acad Dermatol 2019;81(1):91–101.
14. Venanzio V, Galgani I, Polito L, et al. Staphylococcus aureus skin and soft tissue infection recurrence rates in outpatients: a retrospective database study at 3 US Medical centers. Clin Infect Dis 2021;73(5):1045–53.

Assorted Skin Procedures
Foreign Body Removal, Cryotherapy, Electrosurgery, and Treatment of Keloids

Roland Newman II, DO[a],*, Karl T. Clebak, MD, MHA[a],
Jason Croad, DO[b], Kevin Wile, MD[c], Erin Cathcart, MD[d]

KEYWORDS

- Skin procedures • Foreign body removal • Cryosurgery • Electrosurgery
- Keloid treatment

KEY POINTS

- Primary care physicians will encounter different skin issues in the outpatient setting.
- There exist various different approaches when it comes to addressing various skin lesions.
- Primary care physicians should be aware of various procedural approaches to common skin conditions/lesions.

FOREIGN BODY REMOVAL

Primary care providers are commonly tasked with initial evaluation and treatment of skin and soft tissue foreign body (FB) injuries. Injuries range from uncomplicated splinters, to complicated fish-hook wounds. Many pose significant risk of pain, infection, and disfigurement if not properly treated, and can even be a significant source of litigation.[1,2] Multiple considerations for evaluation, imaging, removal techniques, and aftercare will be reviewed here.

Initial Evaluation and Imaging

Up to 38% of soft tissue FBs are missed by providers in the initial clinical examination in emergency departments.[3] Careful attention should be paid to patient risk factors for infection, the mechanism of injury, and signs of neurovascular compromise. Glass, gravel abrasions, deep punctures, and penetration of sharp fragile objects all place

[a] Department of Family and Community Medicine Residency Program, Penn State College of Medicine, 121 Nyes Road, Suite A, Harrisburg, PA 17112, USA; [b] Department of Family and Community Medicine Residency Program, Penn State College of Medicine, 845 Fishburn Road, Hershey, PA 17033, USA; [c] Department of Family and Community Medicine Residency Program, Penn State College of Medicine, 3100 Schoolhouse Road, Middletown, PA 17507, USA; [d] Department of Family Medicine and Community Health, University of Massachusetts Medical School, 55 Lake Ave, North Worcester, MA 01655, USA
* Corresponding author.
E-mail address: rnewman2@pennstatehealth.psu.edu

Prim Care Clin Office Pract 49 (2022) 47–62
https://doi.org/10.1016/j.pop.2021.10.003   **primarycare.theclinics.com**

patients at higher risk for FB injuries and the need for complicated extraction procedures.[1] Imaging is not required before removal of all soft tissue FBs, but should be considered if diagnosis, depth, or local anatomy requires further characterization. Ultrasound may be used to help localize deeper FBs (minimum 0.5 mm detection size), provide guided analgesia, and support sonographic guided removal.[4] Consultation should be considered based on provider comfort level and experience with specific procedures.

Procedure

Indications/contraindications
Early removal is preferred to reduce the risk of infection and avoid a heightened inflammatory response that would prevent easy removal.[5,6] Roughly 25% of patients with skin and soft tissue FBs will present at least 48 hours after initial injury, making evaluation and treatment more difficult.[7] Indications for removal include pain, desire for improved cosmetics, neurovascular proximity/compromise, functional compromise, and infection.[3,8,9] Contraindications to removal in the primary care setting include close proximity to joints, vasculature, or other vital structures; the need for advanced anesthetic techniques; or the inability to localize the FB.[9] Not all FBs require removal, especially if the risks of removal outweigh the benefits. For example, an uninfected, hemostatic, asymptomatic wound containing a deeply embedded FB of inert material (eg, glass or metal) may not require removal.[10,11] Complications of retained FBs include chronic pain, infection, neurovascular impairment, delayed wound healing, and traumatic tattooing (from implanted debris in the dermis that is not removed before re-epithelialization).[12] Complications of removal are similar, plus the risk of iatrogenic injury or incomplete removal.

Analgesia
Procedural analgesia is recommended if deep exploration or excision is required. Digital nerve blocks are beneficial for finger or toe injuries,[13] or an advanced technique such as an ultrasound-guided posterior tibial nerve block can be considered for FB extractions from the plantar foot.[14]

Superficial technique
Ensure adequate visualization (consider a small incision if needed for complete visualization of the FB). Irrigate if needed before removal in order to avoid further contamination with loose debrisConsider careful skin dissection along the entry point with a hypodermic needle or scalpel to expose enough FB material to grasp the FB.Grasp the FB with forceps and slowly withdraw the object.Carefully inspect and irrigate, ensuring that no fragments of the FB remain.

Deep excisional technique
This should be performed under a sterile technique (**Fig. 1**). If the wound is open, it may need to be extended to visualize the base of the FB and extract all material safely without injuring local structures. For a deeper FB around relatively intact skin, make an elliptical excision around the FB (see **Fig. 1**A), angling the tip of the scalpel toward the center of the area to be excised (see **Fig. 1**B). Use a forceps to grasp the skin and any visible FB, providing upward traction (see **Fig. 1**C). Inspect the wound to ensure complete removal of all foreign material. Irrigate thoroughly. Close the incision with suture or wound adhesives.

Vacuum-assisted extraction
Cut off the tip of a sterile syringe (**Fig. 2**A) and use to apply vacuum pressure to extract FBs in difficult-to-excise areas (**Fig. 2**B, C) (see **Fig. 2**)[15].

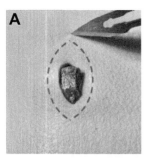
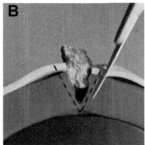
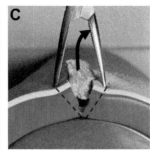

Fig. 1. Deep excisional technique. (*A*) Scalpel used to make elliptical incision. (*B*) Scalpel angle towards center of area to excise. (*C*) Forceps extraction of foreign body.

Fish hooks

These can be particularly difficult, considering the hook may contain multiple barbs that are not visualized under the skin. Three common techniques are used for removal (**Fig. 3**).

- For theneedle cover technique (see **Fig. 3**A), advance an 18- to 20-gauge needle along the embedded portion of the hook until reaching the barb; cover the barb with the needle opening to protect the barb from catching as the needle and the hook are removed together.
- For the advance and cut technique (see **Fig. 3**B), advance the hook in a circular motion until the barb is visualized; cut the barb with a sterile cutting tool. Back the hook out in the reverse direction.
- For the string yank technique (see **Fig. 3**C), loop a string around the curved end of the fishhook. Apply downward pressure to the shank of the hook to disengage the embedded barb. Quickly yank the string in the opposite direction that the needle entered the skin.

Advance and cut technique is used most commonly. Surgical excision should be used as a last resort.[16]

Irrigation

Wounds should be irrigated with saline or tap water after removal to allow mechanical forces to clear debris and bacterial burden from wound. There is no difference between potable water and normal saline in terms of safety or efficacy.[17] Antiseptic solutions should be avoided because of recognized mechanisms for delayed wound healing,[18] with no evidence for benefits over normal saline.[19]

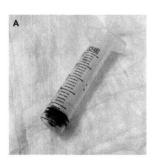
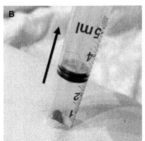
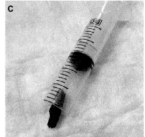

Fig. 2. Vacuum-assisted extraction technique. (*A*) Sterile syringe with tip cut off. (*B*) Syringe placed over location of foreign body. (*C*) Vacuum suction extracts foreign body.

A Needle Cover Technique

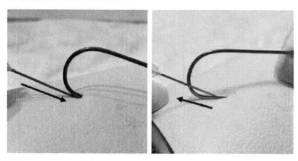

B Advance and Cut Technique

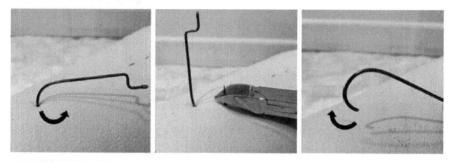

C String Yank Technique

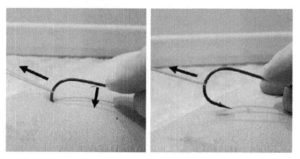

Fig. 3. Fishhook removal techniques. (*A*) Needle cover technique. (*B*) Advance and cut technique. (*C*) String yank technique.

Infection

Antibiotic prophylaxis after FB removal is not generally indicated,[20] except after removal of a retained tooth,[21–23] or in an immunocompromised host. Initiate antibiotic treatment in any wound involving an FB if there is concern for cellulitis or abscess.[22] Recurrent infection despite appropriate treatment should prompt additional imaging for retained FB.[22] Tetanus-containing vaccines should be administered as traditionally indicated per US Centers for Disease Control and Prevention (CDC) guidelines.[24]

CRYOSURGERY

Cryosurgery achieves the destruction of tissue through the application of freezing temperatures.[25–27] In dermatologic procedures, a cryogenic agent is applied directly or indirectly to the skin.[28] The beginnings of cryosurgery can be traced back to the 1800s with the application of a mixture of salt and crushed ice, to the later use of refrigerants, liquid air and oxygen, and carbon dioxide snow.[29] Currently available cryogens include freons, solid carbon dioxide, liquid nitrogen, liquid nitrous oxide, and liquid helium.[25,30] Cryosurgery has become a commonly performed outpatient procedure because of its record of safety, high level of efficacy, low cost, ease of use, lack of an injectable anesthesia requirement, and good cosmetic results.[25,26] Liquid nitrogen has become the cryogen of choice in most clinical applications.[25–27] Effective destruction of malignant lesions requires the lower temperatures achieved through the application of liquid nitrogen through a spray or probe. Liquid nitrogen applied with an applicator is useful in treating benign and premalignant lesions.[27] The mechanism of action includes the direct effects of freezing the cells, osmolarity changes, and the development of local vascular stasis.[31]

Cryosurgery Equipment and Techniques

Cutaneous cryosurgery can be performed with direct application of liquid nitrogen to the skin with a cotton- or synthetic-tipped applicator, liquid nitrogen spray, and cryoprobe. The choice of treatment technique is based on physician training and preference, available clinical resources, and the size, nature, and location of the skin lesion to be treated.

Dipstick technique

The dipstick technique involves dipping a cotton- or synthetic-tipped applicator into liquid nitrogen and directly applying the applicator to the skin lesion. Applicators may be crafted from shaping synthetic material balls and rolling on to the end of an applicator stick.[32] Applicators can also be made from shaping nonsterile 8 inch rayon-tipped swabs. The tip of the applicator may be rolled to a point or hard tail to achieve greater application precision.[33]

Spray technique

Commercially produced spray cannisters apply a fine spray of liquid nitrogen to the skin using nozzles of various shapes and sizes. The spray technique is useful for the treatment of multiple, superficial, or irregularly shaped skin lesions and lesions located on curved body surfaces.[31] The spray is applied with the nozzle perpendicular to the surface at a distance of 1 to 2 cm from the skin lesion. Larger lesions may require spiral, rotary, or paintbrush-type patterns when applying the spray.[25–27] When treating sensitive areas or when spraying in close proximity to nearby structures, a confined technique is performed using a disposable otoscope speculum or folded piece of paper.[25,27,34]

Cryoprobe technique

The cryoprobe technique (also known as contact therapy) is performed by directly applying a cooled metal accessory directly to the skin lesion.[31] The cryoprobe technique is useful for lesions on flat surfaces including the face or eyelids and when there is concern for possible overspray to nearby sensitive structures. A gel medium may be applied between the probe and the skin to facilitate surface contact.

Clinical Applications

Biopsy should be performed prior to cryosurgery when neoplasm is suspected, or the diagnosis is uncertain. The timed spot-freeze technique provides for useful standardization of cryosurgery treatment. The freezing time is based on skin thickness, lesion type, and vascularity.[25–27,30,31] Liquid nitrogen is applied until the resulting ice field encompasses the lesion and establishes the desired margin. Margins for benign lesions are typically 1 to 2 mm, premalignant lesions 2 to 3 mm, and malignant lesions 4 to 5 mm to ensure an adequate depth of freeze.[25–27,30,31,35,36] After the desired margin of ice ball has been achieved, the freeze should be continued to maintain the target margins for adequate freeze time. If more than 1 freeze-thaw cycle is required, complete thaw should be allowed prior to the initiation of the next application (**Table 1**).

Contraindications

Most contraindications to cryosurgery are relative and are generally related to concurrent illnesses. **Box 1** has a list of contraindications.[25–27,30,37]

Complications

All patients should be counseled on complications, and informed consent should be obtained before performing cryosurgery. Avoid overtreatment if cryosurgery is being performed over bony prominences or in areas with superficial nerves. Overtreatment can lead to underlying structure damage and full-thickness skin loss. **Box 2** has a list of potential complications[25–27,35,37,38]

Postoperative Care

Signs of complications, wound care instructions, and healing expectations should be reviewed with the patient after the procedure. Large lesions and malignancies should be washed with soap and water 1 to 2 times a day.[25,30,38] A short course of high-potency topical steroid can reduce large areas of edema.[25,26,31,35] Typical healing time is 2 to 4 weeks for benign and premalignant lesions, but can be up to 14 weeks for larger lesions.[25,26,31]

ELECTROSURGERY
Introduction and Basics

The beginnings of electrosurgery can be traced back to the early 1920s when William Bovie and Harvey Cushing partnered together to pioneer a surgical device that could help control bleeding during surgery.[39,40]

In the primary care setting, electrosurgery can be used for dermatologic procedures – destroying lesions, cutting of skin, and hemostasis.[39,41–44] Advantages of electrosurgery are that blood loss is minimized, and procedural time can be potentially reduced.[44]

Electrosurgery is ideally accomplished through utilization of high-frequency alternating electrical current (AC) by way of a specialized electrosurgical unit (see example: https://www.conmed.com/en/medical-specialties/patient-care/office-based-electrosurgery/hyfrecator-2000/the-hyfrecator-2000-electrosurgical-system) that allows for utilization of different current waveforms/modes for cutting and/or coagulation of tissue at the point of contact.[41–46] Alternating current, as implied, constantly switches direction back and forth. The typical example of AC is that derived from a standard electrical outlet. Lower frequency ACs (those below 1 kHz) typically induce some degree of muscular contraction and tetany.[43–46] However, when AC is applied to tissues at high frequencies, such as 100 kHz or higher, the effects of muscular tetany are minimized to a negligible degree. The ionic movement within cells at such frequencies (typically between 500 and 2000 kHz) generates significant heat, leading to the desired outcomes.[43–45]

Table 1
Cryosurgery indications and techniques

Indication	Usual Number of Freeze-Thaw Cycles	Freeze Time (seconds)	Margin (millimeter of width of ice-ball extending past the lesion)	Expected Number of Treatment Sessions
Benign				
Acne	1	5–15	1	1
Common warts including anogenital and plantar	1–3 (keratinized lesions may require paring, additional freeze and treatment sessions)	10–30	2	1–3
Cutaneous horn	1	10–15	2	1
Dermatofibroma	1	20–60	2	2
Hemangioma	1	10	<1	1
Ingrown nail	1	20–30	2	2
Keloid	1	20–30	2	1–3
Molluscum contagiosum	1	5–10	<1	2
Myxoid cyst	1	20	<1	1
Pyogenic granuloma	1	15	<1	1
Seborrheic keratoses	1–3	10–15	<1	1–3
Skin tags	1	5	1–2	1
Premalignant/Malignant				
Actinic keratoses	1	5–20	1–2	1
Basal cell carcinoma	1–3	60–90	5	1–3
Squamous cell carcinoma	1–3	60–90	5	1–3

Data from Refs.[25–27,30,31,35,36]

Box 1
Cryosurgery contraindications

Absolute
1. High-risk basal or squamous cell carcinoma
2. Melanoma
3. Pathology is required
4. Patient with sensitivity or reaction to cryosurgery
5. Lesions with indefinite margins
6. Patient unable to accept possibility of pigment changes

Relative
1. Cold urticaria or intolerance
2. Agammaglobulinemia
3. Cryoglobulinemia
4. Cryofibrinogenemia
5. Impaired vascular supply
6. Multiple myeloma
7. Pyoderma gangrenosum
8. Raynaud disease
9. Unexplained blood dyscrasia
10. Immunosuppression

Caution should be taken
1. Anticoagulant use
2. Dark-skinned patients
3. Blistering disorders
4. Infants
5. Older patients
6. Sensory loss
7. Irradiated or sun-damaged skin
8. Treatment over bony prominences or areas with superficial nerves

Data from Refs.[25–27,30,37]

Techniques/Indications

The major modalities of dermatologic electrosurgery discussed here are electrofulguration, electrodessication, electrocoagulation, and electrosection. In all such circumstances, the treatment electrode remains cold, while the body acts as the conductor for electrical current.[43] The area treated should be appropriately cleaned and then anesthetized locally with xylocaine, with or without epi, or topical EMLA cream.[41] Basic postprocedure care instructions are provided.

Descriptions of each modality are followed by clinical indications in **Table 2**. In each case, various terminal tips may be used depending on the situation.

Electrodessication

This method involves the electrosurgical terminal coming into direct contact with the skin.[43–46] (**Fig. 4**)When the tissue is heated slowly, water content becomes vaporized, leading to a drying process of the tissue involved.[44] Most damage is confined to the epidermal layer and usually results in little to no scarring.

Electrocoagulation

This primarily occurs when the terminal meets the tissue and heats it to below its boiling point. As a result, the tissue then thermally denatures (see **Fig. 4**). This technique, as it implies, is useful in controlling bleeding during procedures.[43,44,46] Once

> **Box 2**
> **Complications of cryosurgery**
>
> Immediate
> 1. Bleeding
> 2. Blistering
> 3. Edema
> 4. Headache
> 5. Nitrogen emphysema
> 6. Pain
> 7. Paresthesia
> 8. Vasovagal syncope
>
> Delayed
> 1. Bleeding
> 2. Granulation tissue
> 3. Infection
> 4. Tendon rupture
> 5. Ulceration
>
> Prolonged
> 1. Sensation changes
> 2. Hyperpigmentation
> 3. Hypertrophic scarring
> 4. Milia
> 5. Pyogenic granuloma
>
> Permanent
> 1. Alopecia
> 2. Atrophy
> 3. Cartilage necrosis
> 4. Hypopigmentation
> 5. Ectropion
>
> *Data from* Refs.[25,26,30,35,37,38]

tissue becomes coagulated, it develops increased resistance to electricity compared with that of normal skin, thereby limiting the amount of damage done.

Electrofulguration
This is primarily a subvariety of electrodessication and produces superficial tissue destruction.[43–46] (**Fig. 5**) In this method, the terminal is held near to but not directly touching the skin. The high-voltage current can overcome the small gap between the terminal and the skin via a spark, and this spark produces superficial tissue desiccation and carbonization.[45]

Electrosection
The focused application of electrical current results in a rapid increase in the temperature of the tissue (above the boiling point), leading to explosive vaporization of water content in the tissue contacting the electrode.[43–46] (**Fig. 6**) Tissue fragmentation results, and the electrode can pass through the tissue. This is the basic premise behind cutting in electrosurgery.[43,44] Because most of the electrical energy is dissipated during the vaporization process, there is minimal damage to proximal tissues.[43]

Care Points and Considerations

Burns/shocks
Faulty application of the electrode can concentrate electric current enough that it could lead to electrical burns. Fortunately, burns during electrosurgery for

Table 2
Clinical indications and modalities

Indication	Modality			
	Electrodessication	Electrocoagulation	Electrofulguration	Electrosection
Acrochordon	x	x		x
Verruca	x	x	x	
Cherry angiomas	x	x		
Molluscum	x	x	x	
BCC or other small nonmelanotic skin cancers (NMSC)	x	x		
Seborrheic keratoses			x	
Pyogenic granulomas		x		
Pyoderma gangrenosum		x		
Keloids				x
Rhinophyma				x
Certain nevi				x

Data from Refs.[41,43,44,47–50]

dermatologic procedures are rare and more often seen in the surgical literature.[43,46] Shocks can be minimized by avoiding or breaking contact with the patient during application of the electrical current and using an outlet that has a 3-pronged grounding capability.[41,43,51]

Pacemakers, ICD, and cochlear implants
The potential for interference should be considered in patients with pacemakers, implantable cardioverter-defibrillator units, and cochlear implants when electing to choose an electrosurgical method. While data suggest that for most dermatologic procedures the likelihood of complications is low in these individuals, the application of electrosurgical methods should be adapted to each clinical scenario accordingly.[41–43,52,53]

Smoke plume and infection
If the lesion being operated on potentiates the risk of smoke exposure to human papilloma virus (HPV)-associated lesions, proper eye protection, masking, and smoke evacuation should be utilized. Additionally, electrode tips should be replaced or disposed of after each patient, as there is no heat-related sterilization effect of the tip due to the nature of the tip remaining cold during the procedure.[41,43,54–56]

TREATMENT OF KELOIDS

Keloids result from an abnormal response to injury resulting in excess production of collagen and abnormal scar formation extending beyond the wound borders.[57,58] Although benign, keloids can be cosmetically undesirable and painful/pruritic. Keloids

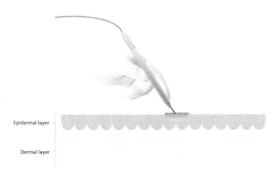

Epidermal layer

Dermal layer

Fig. 4. Electrodessication/electrocoagulation.

are difficult to treat and have a high recurrence rate.[57,58] High-quality research is lacking on the best methods of treatment, as many studies to date have small sample size, high risk for bias, and difficult with blinding treatment methods. Common options for prevention and treatment are described.

Risk Factors and Counseling

Individuals with a history of keloids are at highest risk for recurrence. Dark skin types, younger age, and family history are strong risk factors.[57,58] Certain body areas (sternum, face, ears) and types of injuries (burns) are higher risk also, but any trauma can induce formation (eg, lacerations, piercings, vaccinations, or surgery).[57,58] It is important to counsel patients at high risk prior to procedures on the risks and options for prevention. There is no single best option for treatment, and most are suboptimal for patients with high recurrence. Combination therapies typically offer the best results for patients.[58,59]

Therapy Options

Onion extract
Onion extract is widely available over the counter and at low cost; however, most trials on effectiveness have examined impacts on postsurgical scarring, without a specific analysis of keloid formation. A recent prospective randomized controlled trial (RCT)

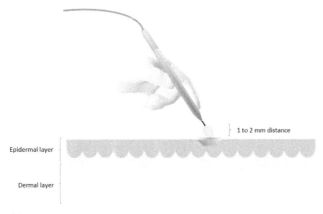

1 to 2 mm distance

Epidermal layer

Dermal layer

Fig. 5. Electrofulguration.

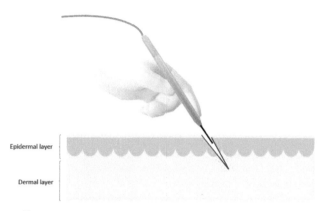

Epidermal layer

Dermal layer

Fig. 6. Electrosection.

examined silicone sheets containing onion extract compared with plain sheets for surgical wounds and found no difference in rates of keloid formation.[60]

Silicone sheeting
The mechanism of silicone sheeting is unknown but hypothesized to be increased moisture and temperature over the wound. Sheets are available over the counter but can be expensive. A recent Cochrane review concluded that evidence for use as monotherapy is weak, with poor regression rates when used for established scars as monotherapy. There is slightly stronger evidence for use for prevention after injuries.[61] Sheeting can be started once the epidermal skin is healed, at least 2 weeks after wound.[59,61,62] Recommendation is to wear sheets 12 to 24 hours per day for at least 2 to 3 months.[61,62] For established keloids, treatment can be longer. The most common adverse event is local irritation, which usually resolves, so treatment is an overall low-risk option.[61]

Pressure dressing
Pressure dressings after procedures can be helpful for prevention but need to be maintained for at least 12 weeks, preferably more than 6 months, to see benefits.[59,63] Reviews have concluded overall low effectiveness, but low risk, so they may be helpful as an adjunct therapy.[59,63] Recommended pressure is approximately 20 mm Hg.[59] Pressure earrings may be helpful after piercings for patients at high risk.[57,59]

Corticosteroid injections
These are proposed to improve keloid scars through anti-inflammatory and antimitotic effects.[64] Multiple RCTs have shown improvement in scar height, pliability, pruritus, erythema, and pain.[59,63,64] Intralesional injections can be performed in primary care offices with relatively low cost. Triamcinolone is the most common steroid used and studied, but methylprednisolone, dexamethasone, or hydrocortisone could be used depending on availability.[61,62] Most studies examined injections of 10 to 40 mg triamcinolone.[63,64] Most protocols suggest injection every 4 to 6 weeks. Regression rates have been estimated at 50% to 100% after 1 year.[63,64] Adverse effects include hypopigmentation, steroid acne, and systemic effects such as hyperglycemia, and pain.[63]

Cryotherapy
Both close spray/contact methods have been used for cryotherapy treatment but have lower efficacy compared with intralesional needle cryotherapy devices.[59,64] External

delivery methods have high rate of hypopigmentation.[64] Cryotherapies are widely available in primary care offices, which makes it a good option in resource-poor settings.[57] This therapy may be most useful for small lesions in noncosmetically sensitive areas.

Laser therapies and radiotherapy

Several options for laser therapies are available. Laser therapies in general have high rates of regression at 6 months but high rates of recurrence at 12 to 24 months.[64] A combination of intralesional corticosteroids and laser therapies appears to be extremely effective at preventing recurrence in small trials.[64,65] Adverse effects include pain, pruritus, hypopigmentation, blistering, and purpura.[59,64] Multiple treatments are required, and it may be difficult to access specialists that provide such services. Radiotherapies are rarely used due to side effects and treatment areas are often high risk for future cancers.[59,64] Advancements in technologies have decreased the risks, and these therapies may remain a good option for patients with significant lesions.

Surgical excision

Surgical excision has been shown to have excellent short-term outcomes; however, because excision creates a new wound, the recurrence rates are estimated at 45% to 100% when used as monotherapy, and it is not recommended unless used in combination with other modalities.[64] Low tension on wound closure should be used to help prevent recurrence.

Methods under investigation

Stem cell therapies, bleomycin, verapamil, angiotensin-converting enzyme inhibitors, interferon, and botulinum toxin A are among emerging treatment therapies.[58,59,64,66] Many have active trials ongoing and will hopefully provide broader treatment options.

CLINICS CARE POINTS

- Keloids are difficult to treat, and high-risk patients should be counseled before procedures.
- Corticosteroid injections, silicone sheeting, pressure dressings, and cryotherapy are reasonable first line treatment options in primary care and are more likely to be efficacious used in combination.
- When considering electrosurgery for a patient, it is important to determine patient history of implanted devices such as pacemakers, ICD's, or cochlear implants due to potential for interference with the functioning of such devices.
- Biopsy should be performed prior to cryosurgery if neoplasm is suspected or diagnosis is uncertain.

DISCLOSURE

The authors have nothing to disclose.

REFERENCES

1. Pfaff JA, Moore GP. Reducing risk in emergency department wound management. Emerg Med Clin North Am 2007;25(1):189–201.
2. Karcz A, Korn R, Burke MC, et al. Malpractice claims against emergency physicians in Massachusetts: 1975-1993. Am J Emerg Med 1996;14(4):341–5.

3. Anderson MA, Newmeyer WL, Kilgore ES. Diagnosis and treatment of retained foreign-bodies in the hand. Article. Am J Surg 1982;144(1):63–7.

4. Rooks VJ, Shiels WE, Murakami JW. Soft tissue foreign bodies: A training manual for sonographic diagnosis and guided removal. Article. J Clin Ultrasound 2020; 48(6):330–6.

5. Ebrahimi A, Radmanesh M, Rabiei S, et al. Surgical removal of neglected soft tissue foreign bodies by needle-guided technique. Iranian J Otorhinolaryngol 2013; 25(70):29–36.

6. Hollander JE, Singer AJ, Valentine SJ, et al. Risk factors for infection in patients with traumatic lacerations. Acad Emerg Med 2001;8(7):716–20.

7. Levine MR, Gorman SM, Young CF, et al. Clinical characteristics and management of wound foreign bodies in the. Am J Emerg Med 2008;26(8):918–22.

8. Skinner E, Morrison C. Wound foreign body removal. StatPearls Publishing. Available at: https://www.ncbi.nlm.nih.gov/books/NBK554447/. Accessed April 12, 2021.

9. Rupert J, Honeycutt JD, Odom MR. Foreign bodies in the skin: evaluation and management. Am Fam Physician 2020;101(11):740–7.

10. Kara MI, Polat HB, Ay S. Penetrated shotgun pellets: a case report. Eur J Dent 2008;2(1):59–62.

11. Winland-Brown JE, Allen S. Diagnosis and management of foreign bodies in the skin. Adv Skin Wound Care 2010;23(10):471–6.

12. Siemers F, Mauss KL, Liodaki E, et al. Accidental inclusions following blast injury in esthetical zones: ablation by a hydrosurgery system. Eplasty 2012;12:e33.

13. Napier A, Howell D, Taylor A. Digital nerve block. StatPearls Publishing. Available at: https://www.ncbi.nlm.nih.gov/books/NBK526111/. Accessed April 13, 2021.

14. Moake MM, Presley BC, Barnes RM. Ultrasound-guided posterior tibial nerve block for plantar foot foreign body removal. Review. Pediatr Emerg Care 2020; 36(5):262–5.

15. Albayati WK, Farhan N, Jasim AK, et al. The utility of a novel vacuum-assisted foreign body extraction technique from wounds. JPRAS Open 2021;27:27–33.

16. Patey C, Heeley T, Aubrey-Bassler K. Fishhook injury in Eastern Newfoundland: retrospective review. Can J Rural Med 2019;24(1):7–12.

17. Svoboda SJ, Owens BD, Gooden HA, et al. Irrigation with potable water versus normal saline in a contaminated musculoskeletal wound model. J Trauma 2008; 64(5):1357–9.

18. Thomas GW, Rael LT, Bar-Or R, et al. Mechanisms of Delayed Wound Healing by Commonly Used Antiseptics. J Trauma-Injury Infect Crit Care 2009;66(1):82–91.

19. Atiyeh BS, Dibo SA, Hayek SN. Wound cleansing, topical antiseptics and wound healing. Int Wound J 2009;6(6):420–30.

20. Lane JC, Mabvuure NT, Hindocha S, et al. Current concepts of prophylactic antibiotics in trauma: a review. Open Orthop J 2012;6:511–7.

21. Ellis R, Ellis C. Dog and Cat Bites. Am Fam Physician 2014;90(4):239–43.

22. Stevens DL, Bisno AL, Chambers HF, et al. Executive summary: practice guidelines for the diagnosis and management of skin and soft tissue infections: 2014 Update by the Infectious Diseases Society of America. Clin Infect Dis 2014;59(2):147–59.

23. Singer AJ, Dagum AB. Current management of acute cutaneous wounds. N Engl J Med 2008;359(10):1037–46.

24. Liang JL, Tiwari T, Moro P, et al. Prevention of pertussis, tetanus, and diphtheria with vaccines in the United States: recommendations of the Advisory Committee on Immunization Practices (ACIP). MMWR Recomm Rep 2018;67(2):1–44.

25. Clebak KT, Mendez-Miller M, Croad J. Cutaneous cryosurgery for common skin conditions. Am Fam Physician 2020;101(7):399–406.
26. Zimmerman EE, Crawford P. Cutaneous cryosurgery. Am Fam Physician 2012; 86(12):1118–24.
27. Andrews MD. Cryosurgery for common skin conditions. Am Fam Physician 2004; 69(10):2365–72.
28. Drake LA, Ceilley RI, Cornelison RL, et al. Guidelines of care for actinic keratoses. Committee on Guidelines of Care. J Am Acad Dermatol 1995;32(1):95–8.
29. Cooper SM, Dawber RP. The history of cryosurgery. J R Soc Med 2001;94(4): 196–201.
30. Graham GF. Cryosurgery. Clin Plast Surg 1993;20(1):131–47.
31. Kuflik EG. Cryosurgery updated. J Am Acad Dermatol 1994;31(6):925–44.
32. Orengo I, Salasche SJ. Surgical pearl: the cotton-tipped applicator–the ever-ready, multipurpose superstar. J Am Acad Dermatol 1994;31(4):658–60.
33. Simon CAMD. A simple and accurate cryosurgical tool for the treatment of benign skin lesions: the "hard tail" dip-stick. J Dermatol Surg Oncol 1986;12(7):680–2.
34. Abide JM. Surgical pearl: readily available cryosurgery shield. J Am Acad Dermatol 2004;51(5):809.
35. Thai KE, Sinclair RD. Cryosurgery of benign skin lesions. Australas J Dermatol 1999;40(4):175–84 [quiz: 185-186].
36. Cooper C. Cryotherapy in general practice. Practitioner 2001;245(1628):954–6.
37. Cook DK, Georgouras K. Complications of cutaneous cryotherapy. Med J Aust 1994;161(3):210–3.
38. Drake LA, Ceilley RI, Cornelison RL, et al. Committee on guidelines of care; task force on cryosurgery. guidelines of care for cryosurgery. J Am Acad Dermatol 1994;31(4):648–53.
39. Marrero K, Fingeret A. The innovator of electrosurgery. J Craniofac Surg 2019; 30(7):1936–7.
40. Meeuwsen F, Guédon A, Arkenbout E, et al. The art of electrosurgery: trainees and experts. Surg Innov 2017;24(4):373–8.
41. Hainer BL. Electrosurgery for the skin. Am Fam Physician 2002;66(7):1259–66 [Erratum appears in Am Fam Physician 2002; 66(12):2208].
42. Taheri A, Mansoori P, Sandoval LF, et al. Electrosurgery: part II. Technology, applications, and safety of electrosurgical devices. J Am Acad Dermatol 2014; 70(4):607.e1–12.
43. Soon S, Washington C. Surgery of the skin. Philadelphia (PA): Elsevier Mosby; 2005. p. 177–90.
44. Taheri A, Mansoori P, Sandoval LF, et al. Electrosurgery: part I. Basics and principles. J Am Acad Dermatol 2014;70(4):591.e1-14.
45. Brill A. Electrosurgery: principles and practice to reduce risk and maximize efficacy. Obstet Gynecol Clin North Am 2011;38(4):687–702.
46. Gallagher K, Dhinsa B, Miles J. Electrosurgery. Surgery (Oxford) 2011; 29(2):70–2.
47. Kim J, Kozlow J, Mittal B, et al. Guidelines of care for the management of cutaneous squamous cell carcinoma. J Am Acad Dermatol 2018;78(3):560–78.
48. Lansbury L, Leonardi-Bee J, Perkins W, et al. Interventions for non-metastatic squamous cell carcinoma of the skin. Cochrane Database Syst Rev 2010.
49. Blixt E, Nelsen D, Stratman E. Recurrence rates of aggressive histologic types of basal cell carcinoma after treatment with electrodesiccation and curettage alone. Dermatol Surg 2013;39(5):719–25.

50. González L, Herrera H, Motta A. Electrosurgery for the treatment of moderate or severe rhinophyma. Actas Dermo-Sifiliográficas (English edition) 2018;109(4): e23–6. https://doi.org/10.1016/j.adengl.2018.03.002.
51. Arefiev K, Warycha M, Whiting D, et al. Flammability of topical preparations and surgical dressings in cutaneous and laser surgery: a controlled simulation study. J Am Acad Dermatol 2012;67(4):700–5.
52. Weyer C, Siegle R, Eng G. Investigation of hyfrecators and their in vitro interference with implantable cardiac devices. Dermatol Surg 2012;38(11):1843–8.
53. Voutsalath M, Bichakjian C, Pelosi F, et al. Electrosurgery and implantable electronic devices: review and implications for office-based procedures. Dermatol Surg 2011;37(7):889–99.
54. Gloster H, Roenigk R. Risk of acquiring human papillomavirus from the plume produced by the carbon dioxide laser in the treatment of warts. J Am Acad Dermatol 1995;32(3):436–41.
55. Lewin J, Brauer J, Ostad A. Surgical smoke and the dermatologist. J Am Acad Dermatol 2011;65(3):636–41.
56. Yonan Y, Ochoa S. Impact of smoke evacuation on patient experience during Mohs surgery. Dermatol Surg 2017;43(11):1363–6.
57. Juckett G, Hartman-Adams H. Management of keloids and hypertrophic scars. Am Fam Physician 2009;80(3):253–60.
58. Betarbet U, Blalock TW. Keloids: a review of etiology, prevention, and treatment. J Clin Aesthet Dermatol 2020;13(2):33–43.
59. Kim SW. Management of keloid scars: noninvasive and invasive treatments. Arch Plast Surg 2021;48(2):149–57.
60. Pangkanon W, Yenbutra P, Kamanamool N, et al. A comparison of the efficacy of silicone gel containing onion extract and aloe vera to silicone gel sheets to prevent postoperative hypertrophic scars and keloids. J Cosmet Dermatol 2021; 20(4):1146–53.
61. Tian F, Jiang Q, Chen J, et al. Silicone gel sheeting for treating keloid scars. Cochrane Database Syst Rev 2021;9(9):CD013357.
62. O'Brien L, Jones DJ. Silicone gel sheeting for preventing and treating hypertrophic and keloid scars. Cochrane Database Syst Rev 2013;2013(9):CD003826.
63. Wong TS, Li JZ, Chen S, et al. the efficacy of triamcinolone acetonide in keloid treatment: a systematic review and meta-analysis. Front Med (Lausanne) 2016; 3:71.
64. Ojeh N, Bharatha A, Gaur U, et al. Keloids: current and emerging therapies. Scars Burn Heal 2020;6. 2059513120940499.
65. Alexander S, Girisha BS, Sripathi H, et al. Efficacy of fractional CO2 laser with intralesional steroid compared with intralesional steroid alone in the treatment of keloids and hypertrophic scars. J Cosmet Dermatol 2019;18(6):1648–56.
66. Mohammadi AA, Parand A, Kardeh S, et al. Efficacy of topical enalapril in treatment of hypertrophic scars. World J Plast Surg 2018;7(3):326–31.

Nail and Foot Procedures

Justin Bailey, MD[a,b],*

KEYWORDS

- Toenail removal • Onychomycosis • Sublingual hematoma plantar wart • Corns
- Blisters

KEY POINTS

- Ingrown toenails can be managed with several alternatives including soaking the feet and allowing the nail plate to grow out, wedge resection, and toenail plate removal.
- Corns and calluses are common problems that are usually resolved by removing the friction-inducing source (ex ill-fitting shoes). Removing the thickened skin over the corns and calluses will often produce pain relief results.
- Blisters are common overuse injuries, and can be prevented with a focused effort on reducing the shearing forces inside the shoes. When needed they can be drained.
- Warts are effectively treated with multiple modalities, including salicylic acid, cryotherapy, candida, or measles antigens.

TOENAIL CARE

Introduction

Disorders of the toenail can be extremely problematic for the patient. Common reasons to consider removal of the toenail include onychomycosis, ingrown toenail (onychocryptosis), trauma resulting in repair of the nail plate or nail bed, or subungual hematoma or blistering.[1] In addition, pain as a result of abnormal growth, such as hypertrophic, incurved, or pincer nails, may warrant intervention.

Anatomy

The nail plate is the hard portion of the nail and the most visible, abutted on each side by the proximal and lateral nail fold. The hyponychium is located just under the distal edge of the nail plate (**Fig. 1**). The nail plate itself is generated from germinative epithelium or matrix located below the proximal nail fold and occasionally observed in the proximal portion on the nail bed (the lunula) where keratinocytes differentiate to form the nail plate. The nail grows out of the matrix and adheres to the vascular nail bed and ultimately separates at the hyponychium.[2]

[a] Family Medicine Residency of Idaho, Boise, ID, USA; [b] Department of Family Medicine, University of Washington School of Medicine
* 5808 N Cape Arago Place, Garden City, ID 83714.
E-mail address: Justin.bailey@fmridaho.org

Prim Care Clin Office Pract 49 (2022) 63–83
https://doi.org/10.1016/j.pop.2021.10.010
0095-4543/22/© 2021 Elsevier Inc. All rights reserved.

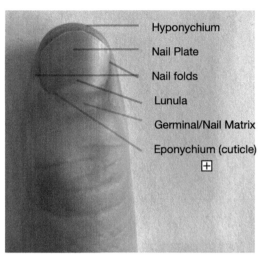

Fig. 1. Toenail anatomy.

Nature of the Problem/Diagnosis

A wide variety of nail problems exist. This article will not discuss dermatologic manifestations of nail pathology beyond those that may benefit from surgical intervention. Although most nail conditions do not require complete removal of the nail plate, a small number of conditions require manipulation of the nail plate. For example, lack of flexibility of hyperkeratotic nails can result in pain at the nail bed. If they are mechanically thinned, or chemically (long-term urea 40%) thinned to a flexible layer, this may lead to resolution of the pain without plate removal.[3] However, reoccurrence is frequent without continued treatment. Toenails that extend past the end of the hyponychium can curve and dig into the skin becoming painful but may be appropriately treated by trimming and not completely removing the nail plate. In patients who have had severe ingrown nails or persistent recurrences, matrixectomy can be considered. The matrix can be ablated surgically, chemically, or with radiofrequency ablation. Partial matrixectomy versus full matrixectomy can be performed depending on the source of the problem.[1]

The most common source of ingrown toenails is inappropriate trimming of the nail plate. Education around trimming techniques and appropriate application can allow for normal nail redevelopment. Nails should be cut straight across the nail plate allowing the edges to grow past the end of the nail ridge[1] (**Fig. 1** shows appropriate nail trimming; **Fig. 2** demonstrates a nail edge below lateral ridges resulting in subungual blisters, now drained). Inappropriate cutting includes trimming the nail too short across the nail bed, or rounding the nail edges below the lateral nail ridges.[1] As ingrown nails are often a result of inappropriate trimming of trauma, matrixectomy is frequently not required (**Figs. 3–9** are a result of poorly trimmed nails). Restrictive footwear and toe trauma (**Fig. 10**) also increase the risk of developing an ingrown toenail.[1]

Patients with limited mobility can have difficulty in trimming nails and may require a clinical visit to assist. Pincer, curved nails, or infected nails (fungal and bacterial) may require complete removal. Ingrown toenails often require partial or complete removal and are the most common presenting nail problem requiring surgery (20% of foot problems)[4]

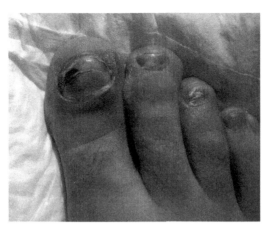

Fig. 2. Subungual blistering. Note the separation of tissue along the superior edge of the nail plate, as well as the swelling along the matrix of the nail. In addition, chronic damage is seen in the second and third toes. The second toe's nail plate is separate from the nail bed.

Surgical Alternatives

Not all ingrown toenails need to be removed. Patients with minor irritation and lack of infection may avoid risks and get a cost-effective, acceptable benefit from a nonsurgical approach. Optimizing footwear to avoid pressure on an ingrown toenail, warm water soaks daily-bid for 10 to 20 minutes with gently working skin away from the

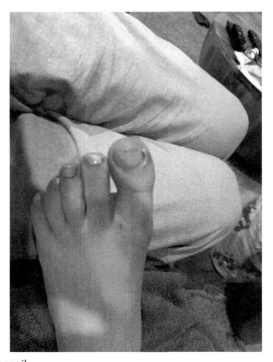

Fig. 3. Ingrown toenail.

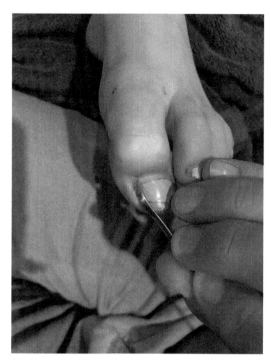

Fig. 4. Single pass with Freer speculum to remove the cuticle.

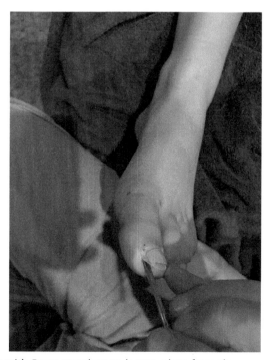

Fig. 5. Single pass with Freer speculum to loosen plate from the area of pressure on the ingrown nail.

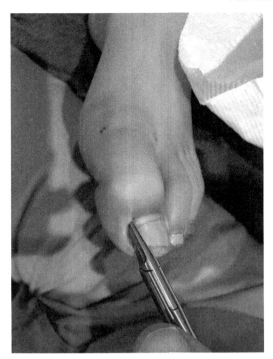

Fig. 6. Nail nipper passed completely to the base of the nail plate. Care is being taken not to injure the cuticle when the nail is cut. Ideally, this is done in a single cut to minimize retained pieces of the plate below the cuticle.

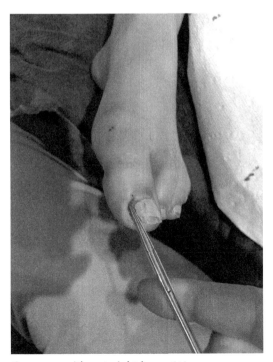

Fig. 7. Wedge resection grasp with a straight hemostat.

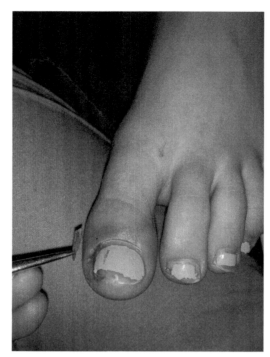

Fig. 8. Wedge resection removed; wedge inspected to make sure all of the nail plate is present.

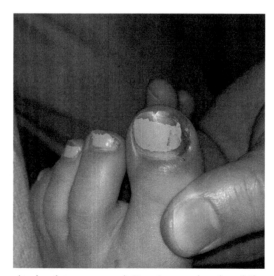

Fig. 9. Nail after wedge has been removed. Dressing can be placed if needed for pain control. Bleeding can be controlled with topical hemostatic agents such as aluminum chloride or silver nitrate.

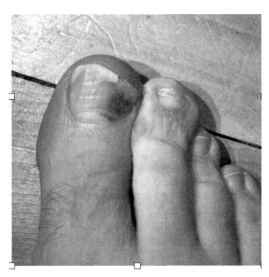

Fig. 10. Subungual bruising from improper footwear.

ingrown toe, and application of a steroid cream for 2 to 14 days can be appropriate nonsurgical approaches.[5] In addition, an approach of placing a bridge or guttural splint under the affected nail edge, such as a cotton wisp or dental floss (usually held in place with a cyanoacrylate adhesive [super glue] under an ingrown nail edge), can be helpful (**Fig. 11**).[6,7]

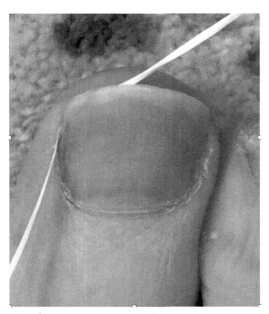

Fig. 11. Example of a dental floss bridge. After the floss is placed, it can be glued in place with a superglue-type product. Cottrell can also be used.

In addition, techniques such as orthonyaxia (using a small metal brace under tension to help direct nail growth) as a conservative measure before nail removal or to help direct nail growth after a partial removal have shown promise.[8]

A Cochrane review showed that surgical treatments for ingrown toenails were more successful than nonsurgical approaches, and that postsurgical treatments, such as antibiotics, honey, iodine with paraffin, hydrogel with paraffin postrepair, did not reduce infection or improve healing times.[4]

Nail Plate Trimming

Nails that curve off the end of the toe (rams horn nails) can be trimmed with a variety of nail trimmers including toenail clippers, or nail nippers. Nails that are difficult to trim can be soaked in warm water or vinegar-soaked cotton balls can be taped over the nails for 15 minutes before trimming to soften the nail and facilitate trimming. In addition, nails that are thickened or difficult to cut can be ground down with a nail grinder (such as a rotary tool with a grinding bit; see **Fig. 12**).[3] After nails are satisfactorily trimmed, emery boards can be used to smooth off any rough edges.

Preoperative/Preprocedure Planning

Shared decision-making to determine the patient's goals should ultimately lead the discussion on what procedure is performed. In addition, a history and physical should be performed paying close attention to disease states that could increase risks of undesired outcomes. Conditions that may result in diminished blood flow to the extremity include tobacco use, diabetes, peripheral vascular disease, coagulopathy, Raynaud's, autoimmune connective tissue disease, and coronary artery disease should be considered.[9] Patients with diminished blood flow to the digit can be at higher risk of infection, worse pain postprocedure, and poor outcomes. Patients with a history of prosthetic joints and prosthetic heart valves may be at high risk for transient bacteremia resulting in infectious sequelae and should be considered in a preprocedure risk assessment. Also, medicines that can increase the risk of bleeding, such as aspirin, NSAIDs, and anticoagulants, should be assessed in addition to allergies to potential procedural exposures (eg, lidocaine, latex).

Physical examination should include assessment of perfusion, skin disorders, or neurovascular compromise.[10–12] For most of the patients presenting to the office, no single condition is an absolute contraindication and shared decision-making

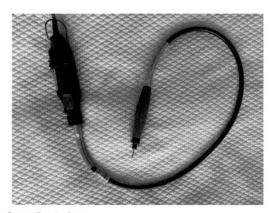

Fig. 12. Example of a nail grinder.

should be used as the provider and patient consider alternative treatments or delaying the procedure (eg, until anticoagulation can be adjusted) in high-risk patients.

Informed consent should include a review of possible risks and benefits including risk of infection and bleeding, expected time for nail regeneration (6 months–1 year), as well as the possibility of nails growing back completely or partially if doing matrix destruction. Antibiotic prophylaxis is not necessary; however, it may be considered in certain situations such as a grossly infected surgical site and a high-risk condition such as heart valve replacement, or recent (last 2 years) artificial joint.[11]

Prep and patient positioning—Most patients are able to have the surgery performed without any premedication. However, the occasional patient may benefit from an anxiolytic medication such as hydroxyzine the night before surgery, or midazolam or lorazepam 30 minutes to an hour before surgery.[13] Patients are usually positioned with the knee bent and the foot flat on the examination table or knee straight with toes pointed up. Patients should be positioned comfortably to minimize movement throughout the procedure.

Surgical approaches can involve partial or complete removal of the nail plate as well as destruction of the nail matrix either chemically or surgically. Wedge resections and full plate removal have similar initial steps and they will be noted in steps of the procedure (see **Fig. 13** for typical toenail removal equipment, **Figs. 14–21** for complete toenail removal, and **Figs. 3–9** for wedge resection).

1. Obtain informed consent and perform preprocedure time-out.
2. Position patients as above so they are comfortable, and the provider has adequate access to the affected foot. Nonpermeable drapes should be placed below the surgical area.

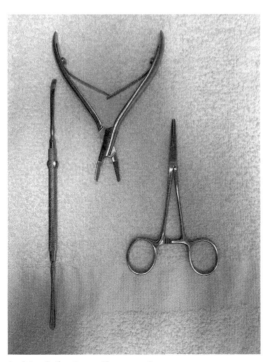

Fig. 13. Typical surgical tools for toenail removal.

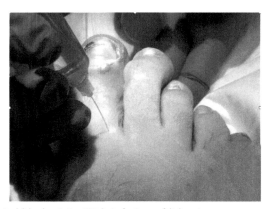

Fig. 14. Step 1 digital block—intra-Web infusion of lidocaine.

3. While observing the appropriate cleaning technique, perform a digital block using 1% or 2% lidocaine, with or without epinephrine[14] (per surgeon's preference). This can be performed by injecting first in the lateral interphalangeal space, passing a 27-gauge 1.5-inch needle (can vary per preference) just lateral to the digit the procedure will be performed and 1 to 3 mL of lidocaine will be injected. Without removing the needle completely, it can then be angled across the dorsal surface of the digit and 1 to 3 mL of lidocaine can be injected. At the far edge of the block, a subcutaneous wheel can be created as an entrance point for the medial injection. Next needle is inserted just lateral to the medial edge of the digit and 1 to 3 mL of lidocaine will be injected (see **Figs. 14–16**). Allow 5 to 10 minutes to pass and check for adequate anesthesia. Repeat digital block or local infusion can be used to complete anesthesia if there are areas where the patient still has sensation.

4. Tourniquets have been used in the past and maybe considered in patients who would be at higher bleeding risk; however, they are not necessary and will allow the provider to localize any area at risk of bleeding before patient leaving the operating suite.

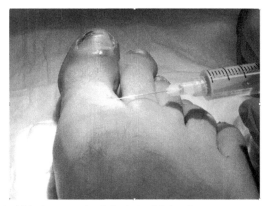

Fig. 15. Step 2 digital block—superior infusion of lidocaine.

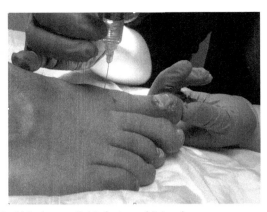

Fig. 16. Step 3 digital block—medial infusion of lidocaine.

5. The toe should be prepped with a cleansing solution such as alcohol, povidone-iodine, or chlorhexidine.
6. A Freer septum elevator (or mosquito hemostat; **Figs. 17** and **18**) should be used to free up the entire nail plate, both superior and inferior, if the entire plate is to be removed. Gentle but firm pressure should be placed under the nail plate and allow the elevator to slide underneath the nail plate until it reaches the cul-de-sac. This is usually located a few millimeters past the end of the nail matrix. Advancement of the septum elevator becomes much easier as it reaches the cul-de-sac. Following this, the septum elevator is placed underneath the nail matrix and the cuticle is separated from the nail plate. This requires firm pressure at first but once the elevator reaches the cul-de-sac, there will be a clear lessening of pressure needed to advance the elevator.
   - If a wedge resection is being performed, a single pass underneath the affected side on both the superior and inferior edge of the plate will be performed, and then a nail splitter/nipper will be advanced along the raised edge to cut the affected edge of the nail off. Care should be taken to avoid damage to the ventral nail matrix (see **Figs. 3–6**).

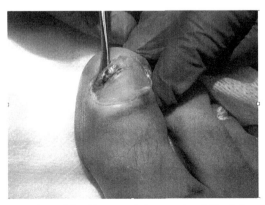

Fig. 17. Nail plate separation with a Freer spatula care should be taken to loosen all the tissues underneath the nail plate.

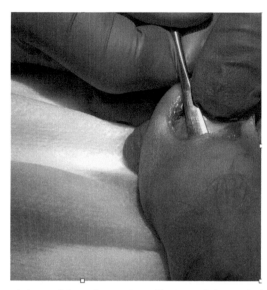

Fig. 18. Loosening of the cuticle and superior adhesion of the nail plate. This should be done into the cul-de-sac of the nail matrix.

- If a complete plate is removed, the entire nail plate, both superior and inferior, will be loosened (see **Figs. 17** and **18**).
7. The nail fragment or plate that is to be removed is then grasped with a straight hemostat or other appropriate graspers. The nail plate should be pulled away from the toe, allowing the nail plate to separate itself from the nail bed. The operator may consider placing a gauze over the nail plate as it is removed to minimize any unintended blood extending beyond the surgical field. The nail plate should come off without tearing or further tissue destruction. If there is an area that is still adherent, the nail elevator can be used to separate the tissue. Lateral rotation without loosening of an adherent nail plate should be avoided to minimize further damage to the nail bed (see **Figs. 7**, **8**, **19**, and **20**).
8. Removed nail plate or wedge should be inspected to ensure the entire plate was removed, as retained nail tissue can further exacerbate pain. Any remaining nail

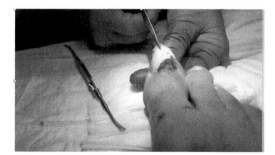

Fig. 19. Removal of the nail plate with a straight hemostat. The nail plate should be grasped and pulled away from the toe, cover the nail plate with a piece of gauze to limit any accidental blood leaving the surgical field. If the nail plate is still in here, then the free speculum should be used to loosen any more adherent tissue.

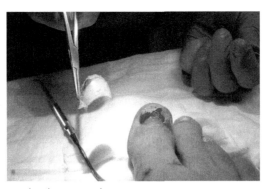

Fig. 20. Nail plate completely removed.

fragments should be removed. Also, lateral nail folds should be examined and a frayed or torn tissue should be trimmed (see **Figs. 7**, **8**, **19**, and **20**).

9. Optional nail matrixectomy can be performed (see the following section).
10. Following the procedure, any areas of bleeding should be addressed. This can be done with pressure with gauze, or other chemical cautery (eg, aluminum chloride solution, silver nitrate sticks) or electrical cautery. This area should then be covered with petroleum jelly/antibiotic ointment and covered with a piece of gauze and secured with an elastic bandage such as coban, adhesive bandage, or elastic gauze. The dressing does not need to be bulky. Patients should be encouraged to wear open-toed or shoes with a wide toe box to the procedure to allow for the comfort with the dressing on discharge (see **Fig. 21**).

Nail Matrixectomy

Electrosurgical
An electrode is placed into the nail bed in the area to be treated. It should be placed in such a way as to minimize damage to the nail bed, keeping the electrode elevated off

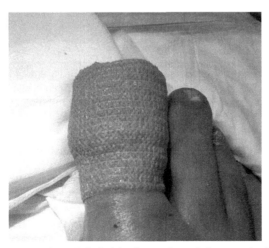

Fig. 21. Dressing postprocedure. A little bit of petroleum jelly on a single 2 × 2 gauze and coban.

the nail bed. The electrode should be activated for a few seconds until a small amount of smoke and searing is heard. This happens very quickly, after just a few seconds. Care should be taken to not over cauterize the area. This will cause prolonged wound healing. Each cautery device should be set to the manufacturer's recommendations. Following this, a petroleum jelly/antibiotic ointment and protective cover should be placed over the surgical area.[4]

Chemical matrixectomy

An 80% to 88% phenol solution can be applied on a cotton-tipped applicator to the matrix. This will be placed into the base of the nail matrix for 30 to 60 seconds, following which the area is rinsed with isopropyl alcohol or saline to flush excess phenol. They should be repeated 2 to 3 times.[4,15–17]

Alternatively, a sodium hydroxide 10% solution can be applied on the cotton-tipped applicator for 60 seconds, following with isopropyl alcohol or saline should be used to rinse the area. The chemical cautery can be caustic to other tissues, so some providers will cover healthy tissues with petroleum jelly before application of chemical cautery. Over application of chemical cautery can result in excessive oozing of tissue as it heals.[4,17]

Recovery and rehabilitation

Pain around the excisions can be expected. Elevation of the affected limb can help reduce swelling and help with pain. Acetaminophen or NSAIDs can help with pain. Dressing with petroleum jelly and a simple adhesive bandage covering can help reduce pain, if the full plate is removed. Pain usually improves over the course of the first week, with exudate resolving in 2 to 3 weeks if a matrixectomy was performed.[1,16]

Outcomes

Wedge resection usually results in rapid improvement in pain. If matrix ablation is undertaken, success rates exceed 95%.[1] Failure of matrixectomy usually is a result of too short of an application of the chemical application.[1,17]

Persistent infection after wedge resection plate removal is uncommon, but if encountered, an antibiotic regimen can be focused on skin flora (eg, cephalexin 500 mg 4 times a day × 5 days).[16]

CALLUSES AND CORNS
Background

Calluses are caused when the foot is exposed to repeated areas of friction or pressure, which result in a thickening of the skin. *Corns* are caused in a similar manner; however, the area of hyperkeratosis has a central core that is often painful to palpation.[18]

Nature of the Problem/Diagnosis

Calluses and corns can appear anywhere on the feet that excessive friction is seen and can become very painful for the patient. Correction of the irritation (such as better-fitting shoes) will often result in the resolution of symptoms.[19] One of the most effective treatment options is determining the cause of the corn or callus and remedying it. Areas of friction or rubbing are often the source of the problem. For example, a hammertoe deformity, pushing the toe into the shoe, will often result in a callus. Tight-fitting shoes can be the source; high-heeled shoes often have a narrow toe box, and the elevation of the heel drives the toes against the sides of the shoe. If these causes can be eliminated, symptoms often resolve, and no surgery needs to be performed. If the area is tender or painful, multiple things can be done to thin the callus or remove the corn.

Treatment Approaches: Reducing Areas of Stress and Friction

Crest pad can be used to reduce a hammertoe deformity. A dental role is placed under the interphalangeal joints of the lesser toe on the plantar aspect. This helps straighten the toes while the foot is load-bearing.[20,21]

Therapeutic padding—A large variety of foam pads, lamb's wool, or silicone sleeves are available over the counter to help reduce friction over corns. If lesions are on the base of the foot over metatarsal heads, commercially available metatarsal pads as well as custom-made metatarsal pads can be created.[21,22]

Shoe stretching can be performed by a shoe cobbler or specialty shoe stores that locate areas of friction and stretch-focused areas. This can be especially helpful around bunions.

Avoidance of poorly fitting shoes. Recommending patients obtain shoes with low rise heels and/or a large toe box, if this is the area of pressure.[19]

Surgical correction can be performed to straighten out hammertoes if conservative methods fail.[23]

Surgical approaches for symptomatic relief

Sharp debridement of hyperkeratotic tissue—Scalpel or chisel blade can be used to pare down the lesion. If a keratin plug is noted, this should be removed. Removal of the hyperkeratotic tissue will almost always provide immediate relief. Presoaking the foot in warm water for 15 to 20 min can help soften skin before sharp debridement. Patients can thin out callous at home with a pumice stone or micrograter after presoaking. It can be difficult to determine if the tissue is hyperkeratotic corn or a wart. If when paring down the lesion, the lesion starts to bleed out of small, dotted blood vessels, it is most likely a wart (see wart section).[24] Although helpful for warts, salicylic acid should be avoided in corns and callouses because of concern for damage to the surrounding tissues, especially in patients with diminished sensation.

BLISTERS
Background

Blisters develop when repetitive shearing trauma occurs at the stratum spinosum. Multiple components go into the development of blisters including skin resilience, moving bone, repetition, and friction. Classically as a foot goes through a repetitive motion (such as running), the skin is held in place between the sock or shoe, and the bone of the foot. This area is unable to disperse the kinetic area of the running motion. The force is then absorbed in the skin at the stratum spinosum. This repetitive shearing results in microtears, which eventually coalesce and filled with serous fluid. After a blister forms, continued forces will result in an unroofing or tearing up the top layer of the blister.[25]

Nature of the Problem/Diagnosis

The most effective way to treat blisters is to prevent them by helping patients understand how they form and working to reduce and dissipate forces that create the blister.[26]

Footwear Fit

The ideal fit creates a shoe that is not so loose that the foot slides around, but not so tight that there is any excessive pressure on focused areas. Running shoes should feel comfortable directly out of the box and do not need to be broken in. Shoes should move well with the foot and not have any areas of noticeable slipping.

Socks

Single or double-layered construction, with moisture wicking properties, is ideal. These include synthetic, or wool blend socks. Cotton, as it becomes wet, tends to become very abrasive and induce blisters. Double-layered construction allows the sock layers to move back and forth dissipating the kinetic energy that would otherwise introduce sheer forces on the foot.

Blister Patches

Smooth patches that go on the insole of shoes or over seams allow socks to slide back and forth, reducing the pinning of the skin that results in shearing trauma. Taping over areas of friction on the foot can also produce a similar effect.

Lubrication

Helps reduce friction between areas of skin such as between toes. Powders can also be used to help reduce friction between feet and socks by wicking away moisture.

Other strategies include pre-exercise taping. This is particularly helpful in the areas that blisters commonly form and are specific to each patient. Orthotics to maintain foot function, skin toughening agents (to increase resilience of skin), removal of calluses before extended activity, antiperspirants to help reduce sweating, gaiters to reduce grit inside shoes and socks, and frequent changing of socks and shoes can also be effective strategies.

Procedure-Draining Blisters

Most blisters do not need to be drained and can be left to heal on their own. Consideration for drainage should include reducing pain secondary to the pressure caused by the blister, or continued activity that may make the blister worse and result in an unroofing of the blister.[26]

1. Clean the skin with an alcohol wipe
2. Use a sterile needle or sterilized pin. An 18-gauge needle allows for a bigger port for drainage and decreased the likelihood of clogging and reaccumulation.
3. Lance the blister 2 to 4 times in different areas. Use pressure from the finger to express the fluid and clean and dry the skin. Dead skin should not be removed. If needles are unavailable, sterile nail clippers or sharp scissors can be used to create a small hole.
4. Area should be covered with antibiotic ointment or petroleum jelly and a sterile bandage. If the activity, which caused the blister to form, is to be continued, addressing areas of friction needs to prevent recurrence or worsening.[26]

SUBUNGUAL HEMATOMA/SUBUNGUAL BLISTERING

Subungual hematoma occurs when bleeding develops below the nail, usually after a crush injury. Subungual blistering develops from prolonged activity and blister development under the nail plate (see **Fig. 2** in complete toenail removal, which shows a drained subungual blister, edges of separation can be seen at the superior border of the nail on the lateral side, and **Fig. 22** shows multiple toes after nail plate removal secondary to subungual blistering). Fluid is trapped between the nail plate and the distal phalanx resulting in compression of the underlying tissue. Patients usually

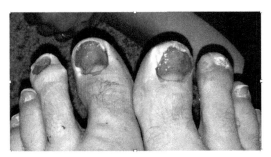

Fig. 22. Toenail trauma after an ultramarathon with multiple toes with subungual blistering requiring plate removal.

complain of severe, throbbing pain. Discoloration or elevation of the nail plate can be noted. Often the digit is swollen.[27]

Procedural Approach—Relief of pressure under the nail plate will ultimately resolve much of the patient's symptoms. A small hole is created in the nail plate to allow drainage. Risks and benefits should be explained and informed consent obtained, including expected damage to the nail plate and possible damage to the nail bed. If there is a concern for a fracture, x-ray should be obtained before drainage. Crush injuries should increase suspicion for a fracture.

1. Handheld cautery units, or a heated paperclip, can be used to burn a small hole through the plate.
2. Once the device is heated, it can be lightly tapped onto the nail plate extending the hole until it reaches the hematoma. Care should be taken to not burn through too far and injure the nail bed. (In addition, an 18-gauge needle or drill bit can be used to bore a small hole; however, there is a potential for nail plate damage, as well as vibratory pressure can result in increased pain.[28] The author's preference is to use a cautery unit or heated paperclip or needle if available.)
3. Once the heated probe has passed through the plate, a small amount of blood will come out of the hole. Gentle pressure around the plate and finger pad can help express the retained fluid. (The patient can do this. Allowing them to be in control diminishes fear around the sensitivity of the nail tip, and is often equally effective to the practitioner doing it.) Most patients have an immediate sense of relief once the pressure is relieved.
4. A consideration for making 2 to 3 holes should be made to minimize the chance of plugging the hole and reaccumulation.
5. If the hole clots, patients can be instructed to soak it in warm water to relieve the clot.

If hematoma involves greater than 50% of the visible nail plate, there should be a concern for nail bed laceration. This is usually seen in a high force crush injury. An x-ray should be done to rule out the fracture. Nail plate injuries require good reapproximation; otherwise, the nail plate will be unable to adhere and will result in a cosmetically unappealing nail plate as well as possible pain associated with poor adhesion. If nail bed injury is suspected, the full plate should be removed and the nail bed evaluated. If a laceration is found, a 6 to 0 absorbable suture should be used to approximate the laceration. Simple interrupted sutures are adequate for repair.[29]

Subungual blisters can be drained in a similar manner; however, if the blister extends to the edge of the nail plate or around the nail plate, passage of an 18-gauge needle into the blister sack is often easier access and can be performed to drain and relieve pressure. If the blister has lifted the entire nail plate off of the nail bed, removal of the nail's plate can be performed, or once the blister is drained, the nail plate will often fall off over the next few weeks.

WARTS
Background

Warts are caused by human papillomavirus, of which there are over 100 different sub-types. Identification of the subtype is not important for treatment. There is a wide variety of treatments that can be used for wart destruction or removal. New warts will often resolve on their own within 2 years, so watchful waiting is an appropriate first step for patients who are agreeable.[30]

Procedural Approach

Pairing down excessive tissue
Most applications will be improved if the wart is pared down before treatment. This can be performed in the office or at home. It is often beneficial to have the patient soak their foot for 5 to 15 minutes in warm water to soften the tissue. A pumice stone or a scalpel can be used to pare down the hyperkeratotic tissue before application of any of the treatments.[31]

Salicylic acid
Can be applied in the office or by patients outside the clinic. Salicylic acid is applied to the wart and covered to maintain contact. Adhesive bandage, adhesive film dressing, or duct tape can be used to keep salicylic acid in contact. Treatments should be continued until the wart clears. If after or 12 weeks, the wart has not resolved, a different method should be considered. Salicylic acid has a 73% cure rate by 12 weeks.[30,32] Limitation with this method includes patient consistency in daily application and difficulties with maintaining adhesive effectiveness to keep application on top of the wart.

Cryotherapy
Liquid nitrogen is generally used to treat warts in the clinic. A spray device or cotton or synthetic tipped swab dipped in liquid nitrogen can be used to create an ice ball and applied over the wart for 10 to 20 seconds. Most practitioners will perform 2 to 3 freeze thaw cycles of 10 to 20 second freezes. Aggressive cryotherapy can also be used (up to 30 seconds per cycle), which produces a higher success rate, however, increases chance of pain and blistering.[28] Patient can return to the clinic every 3 to 4 weeks for repeat therapy if warts have not cleared. After 4 treatments, if the wart has not cleared, there is no additional benefit to continue cryotherapy.[28,33]

Before treatment, informed consent, including potential risks of pain, blistering, tendon or nerve damage, and nail plate damage if treating periungual warts, should be obtained from the patient. Treatment effectiveness with cryotherapy alone is similar to salicylic acid varying between 50% and 70% depending on the trial. Treatment effectiveness is improved if salicylic acid is used in conjunction with cryotherapy.[31,32]

Injectables
Both candida and mumps skin antigens are used to activate a patient's immune response around the wart area. To treat the wart area, clean the area as usual, and inject 0.1 to 0.3 mL of candida or mumps antigen under the wart. A small number of patients may experience itching, burning, or peeling after an injection; however, most tolerate it well. Injections should be repeated every 3 to 4 weeks for up to 3

treatments. Patients can have an allergic reaction, so it is reasonable to consider a trial treatment with 0.1 mL in the forearm before treating patients to assess for tolerance. Patients can have up to 60% clearance with this method.[31]

Duct tape

The use of duct tape for wart destruction has been reported with mixed benefits. Initial studies showed a pronounced effect; however, these results were unable to be repeated in subsequent studies. Currently, there is no support for using duct tape as monotherapy, but can be used as an adjuvant therapy with salicylic acid application.[31,34]

Topical agents

Topical agents such as imiquimod, trichloracetic acid, and cantharidin have limited studies but may prove useful. One small RCT compared imiquimod and salicylic acid with cryotherapy. Patients with imiquimod/salicylic acid had 80% clearance versus 67% clearance at 12 weeks.[35] Higher concentrations of trichloracetic acid applied weekly for 8 weeks appear to be more effective than lower concentrations (80% vs 35% concentration resulted in 47% of patients had a 75% or greater clearance of warts in the 80% group vs 12% in the 35% group).[36] Cantharidin (beetle juice) is not currently available in the United States, but it is used effectively around the world for the treatment of warts. It is a blistering agent that is applied in the office, covered for 2 to 24 hours then washed off. Of concern is the infrequent formation of donut warts (when the central wart clears but then a rim of warts appears around the outside treated edge).[37]

Topical immunotherapy

If none of the above are effective, topical immunotherapy with contact allergens can be performed by an allergist or dermatologist and has been shown to be effective.[38]

Surgical Excision

No randomized studies have been performed evaluating the efficacy of surgical excision; however, reports have been performed with clearance rates upwards of 80%.[38] Multiple different approaches including punch biopsy and elliptical excision can result in removal of the wart tissue. On the base of the foot, consideration should be given to the difficulty of the full thickness excision, failure to heal, and the possibility of permanent painful scars; surgical excision should be reserved for resistant cases with consideration for specialty referral.[31]

Vaccine

The human papillomavirus vaccine has been reported to result in remission of approximately 50% of patients with recalcitrant warts.[39]

SUMMARY

Procedural care for common foot issues is well within the spectrum of primary care providers. These procedures can be added to one's practice, be able to provide timely, effective care for a wide variety of foot conditions.

CLINICS CARE POINTS

- Matrixectomy is not required in all patients with ingrown toenails, but does have the highest success rates at preventing recurrence in patients with multiple repeat infections.
- When treating corns with sharp dissection, keratin plugs need to be removed to resolve pain.

• After a blister is drained if the activity is going to be continued, focused care on reducing shearing friction over the blister site is imperative to limit worsening of the blister.

• Salicylic acid and cryotherapy have similar success rates in wart removal. Candida or measles antigens are good second choices if those fail. Other topical treatments should be third line, and surgery should be saved as a last alternative for patients who fail other treatments. Subungual hematomas that extend greater than 50% of the nail plate should be considered for complete plate removal to evaluate for nail bed laceration in need of repair

DISCLOSURE

The author has nothing to disclose.

REFERENCES

1. Mayeaux EJ, Carter C, Murphy. E Ingrown Toenail Management. Am Fam Physician 2019;100(3):158–64.
2. Haneke E. Surgical anatomy of the nail apparatus. Dermatol Clin 2006;24(3): 291–6.
3. Haneke E, Di Chiacchio N, Richert B. Surgery of the bony phalanx. In: Richert B, Di Chiacchio N, Haneke E, editors. Nail surgery. New York: Informa Healthcare; 2011. p. 149.
4. Eekhof JA, Van Wijk B, Knuistingh Neven A, et al. Interventions for ingrowing toenails. Cochrane Database Syst Rev 2012;4:CD001541.
5. Daniel CR III, Iorizzo M, Tosti A, et al. Ingrown toenails. Cutis 2006;78(6):407–8.
6. Woo SH, Kim IH. Surgical pearl: nail edge separation with dental floss for ingrown toenails. J Am Acad Dermatol 2004;50(6):939–40.
7. Nishioka K, Katayama I, Kobayashi Y, et al. Taping for embedded toenails. Br J Dermatol 1985;113(2):246–7.
8. Hasan Onur Arik MD, al e. Treatment of Ingrown Toenail with a Shape Memory Alloy Device. J Am Podiatr Med Assoc 2016;106(4):252–6.
9. Rich P. Nail surgery. In: Bolognia JL, Jorizzo JL, Rapini RP, editors. Dermatology. 2nd edition. Mosby: Maryland Heights, MO; 2006.
10. Reyzelman AM, Trombello KA, Vayser DJ, et al. Are antibiotics necessary in the treatment of locally infected ingrown toenails? Arch Fam Med 2000;9(9):930–2.
11. H Rosengren, Clare H & S Smith Current Dermatology Reports Update on Anti biotic Prophylaxis in Dermatologic Surgery Current Dermatology Reports, volume1, pages55–63 (2012)
12. DeLauro NM, DeLauro TM. Onychocryptosis. Clin Podiatr Med Surg 2004;21(4): 617–30, vii.
13. Richert B. General considerations. In: Richert B, Di Chiacchio N, Haneke E, editors. Nail surgery. New York: Informa Healthcare; 2011. p. 16.
14. Ilicki J. Safety of epinephrine in digital nerve blocks: a literature review. J Emerg Med 2015;49(5):799–809.
15. Di Chiacchio N, Di Chiacchio NG. Best way to treat an ingrown toenail. Dermatol Clin 2015;33(2):277–82.
16. Peggs JF. Ingrown toenails. In: Pfenninger JL, Fowler GC, editors. Pfenninger and Fowler's procedures for primary care. 2nd edition. Mosby: Maryland Heights, MO; 2003. p. 269–72.
17. Grover C, Khurana A, Bhattacharya SN, et al. Controlled trial comparing the efficacy of 88% phenol versus 10% sodium hydroxide for chemical matricectomy in

the management of ingrown toenail. Indian J Dermatol Venereol Leprol 2015; 81(5):472-7.

18. Thomas SE, Dykes PJ, Marks R. Plantar hyperkeratosis: a study of callosities and normal plantar skin. J Invest Dermatol 1985;85:394-7.

19. Richards RN. Calluses, corns, and shoes. Semin Dermatol 1991;10:112-4.

20. White SC. Padding and taping. In: Valmassy RL, editor. Clinical biomechanics of the lower extremities. St Louis (MO): Mosby; 1996. p. 368-89.

21. Freeman D. Corns and Calluses Resulting from Mechanical Hyperkeratosis. Am Fam Physician 2002;65(11):2277-80.

22. Singh D, Bentley G, Trevino SG. Callosities, corns, and calluses. BMJ 1996;312: 1403-6.

23. Pontious J, Lane GD, Moritz JC, et al. Lesser metatarsal Vosteotomy for chronic intractable plantar keratosis. Retrospective analysis of 40 procedures. J Am Podiatr Med Assoc 1998;88:323-31.

24. Dockery GL, Crawford ME. Cutaneous disorders of the lower extremity. Philadelphia: Saunders; 1997. p. 247-50.

25. Naylor P. Experimental Friction Blisters. Br J Dermatol 1955;67 10:327-42.

26. Vonhof, John, Fixing your feet Wilderness Press Biringham Alabama 2016.

27. Van Beek AL, Kassan MA, Adson MH, et al. Management of acute fingernail injuries. Hand Clin 1990;6:23-38.

28. Skinner Paul. Management of Subungual Hematoma. Am Fam Physician 2005; 71(5):856.

29. Rockwell WB, Wray RC Jr. Nail bed injuries and reconstruction. In: Peimer CA, editor. Surgery of the hand and upper extremity, vol. I. New York: McGraw-Hill, Health Professions Division; 1996. p. 1101-11.

30. King-fan Loo S, Yuk-ming Tang W. Clinical Evidence. Warts (non-genital). 2009. Available at: http://clinicalevidence.bmj.com/ceweb/conditions/skd/1710/1710.jsp. Accessed September 14, 2021.

31. Mulhem Elie, Pinelis S. Treatment of Nongenital Cutaneous Wart. Am Fam Physician 2011;84(3):288-93.

32. Gibbs S, Harvey I. Topical treatments for cutaneous warts. Cochrane Database Syst Rev 2006;3:CD001781.

33. Berth-Jones j, Hutchinson PE. Modern treatment of warts. Br J Dermatol 1992; 127(3):262-5.

34. Wenner R, Askari S, Cham P, et al. Duct tape for the treatment of common warts in adults: a double-blind randomized controlled trial. Arch Dermatol 2007;143(3):30.

35. Stefanaki C, Lagogiani I, Kouris A, et al. Cryotherapy versus imiquimod 5% cream combined with a keratolytic lotion in cutaneous warts in children: A randomized study. J Dermatolog Treat 2016;27(1):80.

36. Pezeshkpoor F, Hashemi B, Yazdanpanah M, et al. Comparative study of topical 80% trichloroacetic acid with 35% trichloroacetic acid in the treatment of the common wart. J Drugs Dermatol 2012;11(11):e66-9.

37. Sterling JC, Gibbs S, Haque Hussain SS, et al. British Association of Dermatologists' guidelines for the management of cutaneous warts 2014. Br J Dermatol 2014;171:696.

38. Kwok CS, Gibbs S, Bennet C, et al. Topical treatments for cutaneous warts. Cochrane Database Syst Rev 2012;2012(9):CD001781.

39. Yang MY, Son JH, Kim GW, et al. Quadrivalent human papilloma virus vaccine for the treatment of multiple warts: a retrospective analysis of 30 patients. J Dermatolog Treat 2019;30(4):405.

Management of Chronic Wounds

Ashley Morrison, MD[a], Charles Madden, MD[b], John Messmer, MD[a],*

KEYWORDS

- Chronic wounds • Venous ulcers • Pressure injury • Arterial ulcers

KEY POINTS

- Venous ulcerations are the most common type of lower extremity wound, resulting from chronic venous insufficiency; diagnosis should include venous duplex ultrasound as well as ankle brachial index to rule out arterial disease.
- Management of venous wounds includes a combination of compression, debridement, exudate control, and treatment of bacterial infection if present.
- Arterial wounds have complex causes requiring multiple specialties for management.
- Pressure ulcers are often preventable by pressure avoidance and management of risk conditions.

 Video content accompanies this article at http://www.primarycare.theclinics.com.

VENOUS WOUNDS

Introduction

Venous ulcerations are the most common type of lower extremity ulcer.[1] Venous ulcers are estimated to affect 1% to 1.5% of the adult population.[2] The overall prognosis of venous ulcers is generally poor, with recurrence rates exceeding 50%.[2]

Chronic venous insufficiency results from ambulatory venous hypertension, defined as a failure to reduce venous pressure with exercise.[3] In a healthy state, the venous valves and muscular pumps of the lower leg limit the accumulation of blood in the lower extremity veins. Peripheral venous insufficiency results when the lower extremity muscle pumps fail, which can result from outflow obstruction, muscle weakness, loss of joint motion, or valve failure.[3]

[a] Department of Family and Community Medicine, Penn State College of Medicine, Hershey, PA 17033, USA; [b] Spectrum Health Big Rapids Hospital Family Medicine, 650 Linden St, Suite 1, #MC350, Big Rapids, MI 49307, USA
* Corresponding author.
E-mail address: jmessmer@pennstatehealth.psu.edu

Prim Care Clin Office Pract 49 (2022) 85–98
https://doi.org/10.1016/j.pop.2021.10.009
0095-4543/22/© 2021 Elsevier Inc. All rights reserved.

Pathologic effects in the skin and subcutaneous tissues such as edema, pigmentation, and ulceration result from chronic venous hypertension, which can also be thought of as sustained venous pressure elevation.[3]

Evaluation

The first step in evaluating venous wounds should be obtaining a comprehensive medical history and review of symptoms. Symptoms that suggest venous disease include extremity pain, burning, aching, throbbing, cramps, heaviness, itching, tiredness, fatigue, and restless legs.[4] Limb dependency usually exacerbates symptoms caused by venous hypertension, whereas rest or elevation relieves them. Risk factors associated with venous disease include age, elevated body mass index, previous venous thromboembolism, family history of varicose veins, episodes of superficial thrombophlebitis, spontaneous venous rupture, prior use of compression therapy, prior venous operative interventions, use of venotonic medications such as horse chestnut seed or butcher's broom extracts, and presence of other systemic diseases associated with leg wounds (such as neurologic conditions such as multiple sclerosis, cardiovascular conditions such as hypertension, metabolic conditions such as diabetes, and autoimmune conditions such as Wegener granulomatosis).[4] On physical examination, telangiectasia, varicose veins, edema, skin discoloration, inflammation, eczema, hyperpigmentation, malleolar flair, **corona phlebectatica** (abnormally dilated veins around the ankle), **atrophie blanche** (white atrophic scar from a healed ulcer),

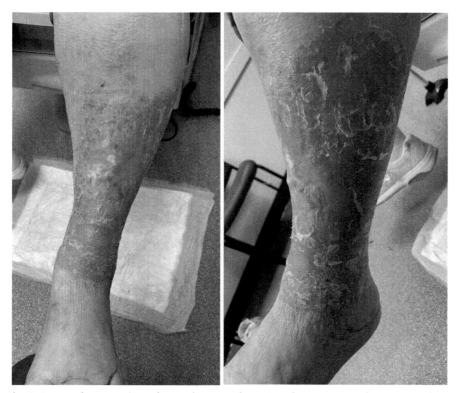

Fig. 1. Venous hypertension. The erythema and crusting due to tissue edema are evident. Note that the foot is free of these changes due to compression from shoes.

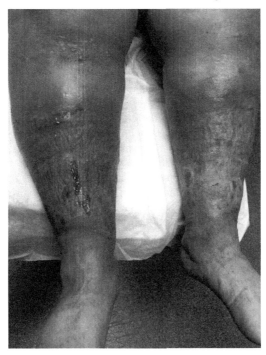

Fig. 2. Hyperpigmentation from chronic stasis. Skin breakdown increases infection risk.

palpable venous cord, tenderness, and induration suggest venous disease[4] (**Figs. 1 and 2**).

On examination, the lower extremity should be palpated for tenderness, induration, edema, pulses, palpable venous cord, and evaluation of ankle mobility. Venous wounds should be measured and documented at every visit to determine baseline and effect of treatment. The measurements should include location on leg, area, perimeter, and depth, as well as a description of wound edge parameters, base quality, drainage, and signs that suggest infection. Serial photographs should be obtained at office visits for comparison if possible. There is no evidence to support routine surface cultures of venous wounds unless there are signs of active infection. These wounds are usually colonized by multiple microorganisms, with Staphylococcus, Pseudomonas, and Enterobacter being the most common pathogens.[5] Signs of infection that would prompt need for culture include fever, leukocytosis, worsening pain, cellulitis, purulent drainage, increased exudate, malodor, discolored friable granulation tissue, biofilm, tissue necrosis, or ulcer progression.[4]

If a venous wound is not responding to standard treatment within 4 to 6 weeks, tissue biopsy is recommended to assess for other causes of ulceration. Biopsies should be obtained from several sites.[4] Patients with recurrent or difficult to treat venous ulcerations may have an increased risk of thrombophilia. This risk is increased in patients with prior thrombosis, family history of thrombotic events, and onset of venous ulcerations before the age of 50 years. It is recommended to initiate a workup for thrombophilia for patients with a history of recurrent venous thrombosis and chronic recurrent venous leg ulcers. This workup should include testing for antithrombin deficiency, protein C and protein S deficiencies, factor V Leiden, prothrombin G20210A, plasminogen activator inhibitor type 1 mutations, hyperhomocysteinemia, antiphospholipid antibodies, and cryoglobulins and cryoagglutinins.[4]

Imaging

Venous duplex ultrasound is recommended as part of diagnostic assessment in all venous wounds to evaluate for both obstructive and reflux patterns of venous disease. Venous plethysmography provides additional venous limb physiologic parameters and may be used if the venous duplex ultrasound is equivocal or for recalcitrant or recurrent venous leg ulcerations.[4]

Approximately 15% to 25% of patients with venous leg ulcerations will also have peripheral arterial disease;[4] therefore, it is recommended that an ankle-brachial index measurement is performed on all patients with venous leg ulcerations. Patients with venous leg ulcerations and suspected venous obstruction (thrombotic or nonthrombotic) should undergo contrast imaging with computed tomography venography or magnetic resonance venography. Diagnosis should then be confirmed by contrast venography and intravascular ultrasound.[4]

Approach

The management of venous wounds involves several key components. Wound bed preparation is undertaken to accelerate endogenous healing and provide a conducive environment for other measures to be effective. The goal is to convert the environment of a chronic wound to that of an acute healing wound through debridement, wound exudate control, and management of surface bacteria. There is little evidence regarding wound cleansing before dressing application; however, the Society of Vascular Surgery recommends routinely cleansing wounds before dressing changes to remove wound exudate and debris that are often present.[4]

There are several different types of dressings that are used in the treatment of venous ulcers. Hydrocolloids (complex multilayer adherent dressings), foams (absorbent dressings), alginates (highly absorbent soluble dressings), hydrogels (amorphous moisturizing dressings), and low-adherent absorptive dressings have been compared in various studies with no dressing type being shown to be more effective as far as number of ulcers healed.[6] Dressings should be chosen based on need for exudate management, clinical response to treatment, and patient comfort. Oral pentoxifylline promotes ulcer healing with and without compression therapy; however, oral zinc is not effective in healing venous ulcers.[7]

Table 1 Types of dressings			
Dressings that Increase Moisture	Dressings that Decrease Moisture	Dressings that Facilitate Autolytic Debridement	Antibacterial Dressings
Transparent films	Calcium alginate dressings	Hydrogels	Silver-based agents (available as hydrogels, alginates, foams, compression garments)
Hydrocolloids	Foam	Films	Polyhexamethylene biguanide
Hydrogel dressings	Hydrofiber	Hydrocolloids	Cadexomer iodine
	Composite dressings		Holyacrylates

Data from Gist S, Tio-Matos I, Falzgraf S, Cameron S, Beebe M. Wound care in the geriatric client. Clin Interv Aging. 2009;4:269-287.

Moisture balance must be maintained in the wound bed, and this can be accomplished with newer generation of wound dressings that increase moisture to wounds that are too dry and decreasing moisture of wounds that are too wet.[8] Dressings are compared in **Table 1**.

There are 6 different methods of debridement: surgical debridement with a scalpel, mechanical debridement with washing solutions and dressings, enzymatic debridement, autolytic debridement with moist dressings or natural agents, and biosurgical debridement with maggots. A 2015 Cochrane Review including 10 randomized controlled trials (RCTs) (N = 715 participants) concluded that there is limited evidence to suggest that actively debriding venous leg ulcers has a clinically significant impact on healing.[9]

It is important to consider anesthesia for surgical debridement of wounds. For debridement, a topical EMLA Cream application provides effective pain relief.[10] If the debridement is to be more extensive, local anesthesia, a regional block, or general anesthesia may be needed.

The Society for Vascular Surgery recommends surgical debridement when there is slough, nonviable tissue, or eschar present in the wound bed (Grade 1 LOE B), with hydrosurgical debridement as an alternative (Grade 2 LOE B).[4] If no clinician trained in surgical debridement is present, then enzymatic debridement is recommended (Grade 3 LOE C). Biological debridement with larval therapy can be used as an alternative to surgical debridement (Grade 2 LOE B).[4]

Compression is an important component in the treatment of lower extremity venous ulcers. Compression bandaging systems are classified as either short or long stretch. Short-stretch systems, such as multilayer or the traditional Unna boot, are most appropriate for ambulatory patients, as they produce higher walking pressures. The Unna boot uses a rigid shell to enhance the calf muscle pump during ambulation. Long-stretch compression systems (ie, single layer or highly elastic) produce higher resting pressure and are indicated in nonambulatory patients. A 4-layer compression system shortens time to healing and is associated with lower adverse event rates and higher quality-of-life scores compared with single-layer systems.[6] However, there does not seem to be a significant difference between 4-layer systems and 2- and 3-layer systems.[6]

The technique for application of an Unna boot can be viewed in (Video 1).

A 2012 Cochrane review of 48 RCTs suggested that compression increases ulcer healing rates compared with no compression.[11] Multicomponent systems are more effective than single-component systems, particularly those with an elastic bandage.[11] Intermittent pneumatic compression may improve healing but data are inconsistent. A Cochrane review found that intermittent compression is better than no compression, but studies vary in quality.[11]

There are contradictory data regarding the treatment of bacterial colonization of venous wounds. Most open ulcers are contaminated, but if signs of cellulitis or colonization, such as, erythema, odor, and purulent drainage are present, healing may be delayed.[12]

Surgical correction of venous hypertension (ie, saphenous stripping) is an option in treatment and prevention of healing of venous ulcers.[6] Intermittent pneumatic compression may be helpful to correct edema in some cases, although chronic compression is better than no compression.[13,14]

In a study, simvastatin, 40 mg, daily in addition to standard wound care and compression was associated with improvement in healing rate and time of venous ulcers.[2]

Arterial and Atypical Ulcers

Ulcers may develop from arterial insufficiency due to atherosclerosis. Poorly controlled medical problems such as diabetes, hypertension, hyperlipidemia, hypertension, and smoking result in arterial narrowing and reduced oxygen delivery to tissues. Although this commonly occurs distally, ulcers can develop in any area with minimal collateral circulation. These ulcers tend to be dry and may have necrotic tissue and eschar present.[15] Ankle-brachial index less than or equal to 0.9 can support a diagnosis of peripheral arterial disease. Doppler studies can confirm arterial insufficiency as well as evaluating the venous system.

Atypical location, appearance, or symptoms or failure to respond to conventional therapy may lead to the suspicion of an atypical ulcer. Other causes to consider include vasculitis, calciphylaxis, pyoderma gangrenosum, or malignancy. A punch biopsy may be needed to confirm the diagnosis.[15,16]

Autoimmune causes are extremely resistant to conventional therapies and may involve immunosuppression, vasodilators, anticoagulants, debridement, hyperbaric oxygen, regeneration activators, and skin transplantation.[16,17] Malignant ulcers may require surgery or other specialized interventions.

Management of these ulcers will typically be a multispecialty process depending on the cause.

PRESSURE INJURY
Introduction

Pressure injuries, previously called pressure ulcers, are damage caused to the skin and underlying soft tissue due to pressure. These usually occur over boney prominences or are related to use of devices such as medical equipment. With the injury, skin integrity can be intact or open. The injury is due to intense and/or prolonged pressure or pressure in combination with shear forces. Location, microclimate, nutrition, perfusion, and comorbid conditions all contribute to the risk of pressure injuries.[18]

Epidemiology

In the United States, pressure injuries affect around 2.5 million people a year in acute care facilities.[19] These injuries, particularly stages 3 and 4, lead to increased medical costs estimated around $26 billion per year.[20] Studies have shown that the cost for treating these injuries have increased over the past decade.[20–22] In addition, the US Centers for Medicare and Medicaid Services do not reimburse for pressure injuries sustained in acute care hospitals.[20] In order to incentivize hospitals to improve patient safety, Centers for Medicare and Medicaid Services developed the Hospital-Acquired Condition Reduction Program, which reduces payments to hospitals who score poorly in categories such as pressure ulcer rate, in-hospital fall with hip fracture, and perioperative hemorrhage by 1%.[23]

The prevalence rates among hospitalized patients vary from 5% to 15% with the highest risk in patients in intensive care unit.[24] National Pressure Ulcer Prevalence Survey from 1989 to 2005 showed pressure injuries were most prevalent in long-term acute care facilities ranging from 23% to 27%, whereas less in acute care and long-term care facilities.[24,25] Data from the 2006 to 2015 surveys showed the prevalence remained elevated in long-term acute care facilities ranging from 28% to 37%. It did show decreased overall prevalence in acute care and long-term care facilities.[26] Patients with neurologic impairments have an increased risk of developing pressure injuries as do the elderly.[24]

Pathophysiology

Prolonged pressure elicits a feedback response, which triggers the body to change positions.[24] When this feedback is impaired, it leads to increased risk for injury from sustained pressure causing tissue ischemia, injury, and can lead to necrosis.[24,27]

Generally, pressure from body weight exerts a downward force on skin and tissue between bony prominence and an external surface. If this pressure is greater than the capillary filling and venous outflow pressures, blood flow is inhibited, which leads to local hypoxia.[24] Sustained pressure for an extended period of time can progress to ischemia and necrosis. Muscle is at increased risk for hypoxia compared with subcutaneous tissue and skin; a pressure injury visible on the skin may indicate the presence of extensive deep tissue injury.[24,27]

Shear and friction forces can lead to disrupted blood flow and injury as vessels are stretched and distorted.[24,28]

Risk Factors

Patients most at risk for pressure injury are those with impaired mobility/activity, sedation, peri- or postoperative immobilization, frailty, or at high risk for friction or shear injuries.[24] These patients are likely to experience prolonged periods of pressure leading to injury.[19,24] Patients with history of pressure injuries or current pressure injuries are at increased risk of forming another. Comorbid conditions that increase risk of pressure injuries include diabetes, poor perfusion, neuropathy, spinal injuries, and severe illnesses. Poor nutrition also increases risk of injuries due to malnutrition.[19] Elderly are particularly vulnerable due to muscle loss and natural skin thinning and other changes putting them at increased risk of shearing forces.[24,29] Moisture and temperature also increase the risk of injury through maceration and skin break down.[19,24,30]

Diagnosis

Pressure injuries can occur anywhere where prolong pressure occurs. They most commonly occur at locations overlying bony prominences, including the sacrum, ischial tuberosity, greater trochanter, heels, and lateral malleolus.[24]

The National Pressure Ulcer Advisory Panel last updated staging guidelines in 2016. Wounds range from stage 1 to 4 (with 4 being the most severe).[18] Wounds can also be classified as unstageable due to debris or eschar preventing full evaluation. The staging of pressure injures are described in **Box 1**.

Prevention

Prevention of pressure injuries involves a multicomponent approach beginning with screening and risk assessment to address preventable causes. There are several available risk assessment tools; the most commonly used tools include the Braden, Norton, and Waterlow scales. Although frequently used, these tools have a low sensitivity and specificity for identifying at-risk patients.[24] Studies have demonstrated that the tools may not be superior to clinical judgment when assessing patients for risk.[24,31] Whether using screening tools or clinical judgment, patients should be screened immediately on admission to an inpatient care facility or regularly in the clinic setting if they have a known risk factor.[19]

The use of multiple therapies and a standardized approach to assessing risk and preventing pressure injuries reduces injury rates.[19,31,32] Health systems should have structured, multifaceted programs aimed at reducing the incidence of pressure injuries.[19,31]

Repositioning is an essential element to pressure prevention.[19,33,34] Repositioning reduces the pressure in one area, allowing decreased length of hypoxia and tissue injury. Traditional recommendations recommend repositioning every 2 hours, but data show that this is not significantly better at reducing pressure injuries compared with repositioning at 3- to 4-hour intervals.[31,33,34] Because of this, repositioning should be based on patient's level of activity, mobility, and ability to move independently. It is

---

Box 1
Pressure ulcer stages

Stage 1: skin will be intact with localized area of nonblanchable erythema. Presence of blanchable erythema or changes in sensation, temperature, or firmness may be seen before visual changes (**Fig. 3**).

Stage 2: there will be partial-thickness loss of skin with exposed dermis. The wound bed will be pink or red, moist, and may be associated with an intact or ruptured serum-filled blister. Adipose tissue will not be present nor will granulation tissue, slough, or eschar (**Fig. 4**).

Stage 3: there will be full-thickness skin loss where adipose tissue is visible. Granulation tissue, eschar, and slough may be present but do not obscure the depth of the wound. Undermining and tunneling may occur. No other structures are visible at base of wound (**Fig. 5**).

Stage 4: there will be full-thickness skin and tissue loss with exposed or palpable fascia, muscle, tendon, ligament, cartilage, or bone within the ulcer. Slough, eschar, tunneling, and undermining may be present but do not obscure the extent of tissue loss (**Fig. 6**).

Unstageable: there is full-thickness skin and tissue loss in which the extent of damage cannot be determined. This is most commonly obscured by eschar or slough (**Fig. 7**).

Deep tissue pressure injury is when intact or nonintact skin is nonblanchable deep red, maroon, or purple discoloration. Pain and temperature variations are often present. The injury may resolve or progress to further tissue lost. These often mark a full-thickness injury (stage 3 or 4) (**Fig. 8**).[14]

---

also important to take into account patient medical conditions, skin integrity, comfort, and pain. It can be beneficial to use alerting systems to prevent missing repositioning events. Patients should be encouraged to sit up in chairs when able for short periods of time.[19]

Monitoring the patient's angle of incline is also important, as increased angles lead to shear and friction forces.[33] Having patients in 30° lateral tilt compared with supine or at 90° lateral positioning decreases pressure injuries.[19,33]

Support surfaces have also been shown to decrease incidence and severity of pressure injuries. These include high-specification foam, bead-filled, and water-filled mattresses and alternating pressure mattresses and overlays.[33] Constant low-pressure and alternating pressure supports reduce the incidence of pressure injuries when compared with standard mattresses.[31,33,35] These supports should be used in the bed as well as with chairs and wheelchairs for patients seated for prolonged periods of time.[19]

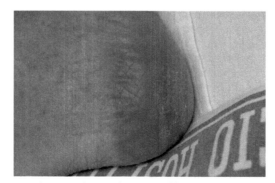

Fig. 3. Stage 1 pressure damage. (*From* Shutterstock)

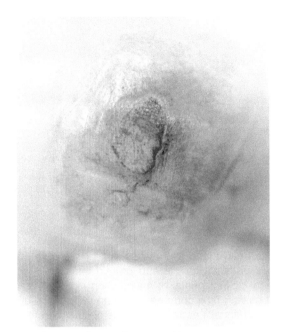

Fig. 4. Stage 2 pressure damage. (*From* Shutterstock)

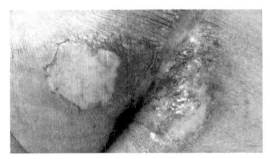

Fig. 5. Stage 3 pressure damage. (*From* Shutterstock)

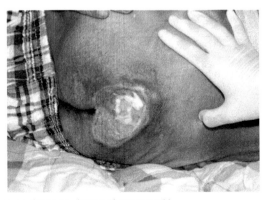

Fig. 6. Stage 4 pressure damage. (*From* Shutterstock)

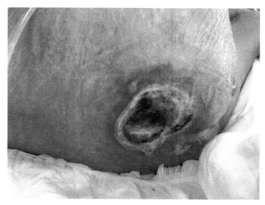

Fig. 7. Unstageable pressure damage. (*From* Shutterstock)

Poor nutrition has been found to increase risk of pressure injury formation. It is important to assess patient's calorie and protein intake as well as recent weight loss when assessing for indications of malnutrition.[19,33,36] Protein supplementation can reduce rate of healing time compared with no supplementation.[37] If a patient is not meeting their nutritional needs orally, enteral and parenteral feeding can be considered. These conversations should include discussing risk and benefits with the patient and ensuring the options are in line with health goals.[36] There is no significant difference between oral and enteral feeding although enteral feeding is less well tolerated.[31] Patients should be provided with 30 to 35 kcal/kg body weight/d, 1.2 to 1.5 g protein/kg body weight/d, and high-calorie diet for patients who are malnourished or at risk of malnutrition to help prevent injury formation.[19,36]

There are many forms of dressings that have been found to help protect the skin from pressure injuries. These dressings mainly help by reducing shear or friction forces on high-risk skin areas.[33] Studies have shown that the use of prophylactic sacral dressings can reduce incidence of pressure injuries more notably in critically ill patients.[8] Dressings should be selected and placed based on the patient's needs.

Treatment

The mainstays of treatment include all of the principles of prevention, specifically off-loading through repositioning, using pressure reducing support surfaces, and providing adequate nutrition for proper wound healing.[33] Additional measures include

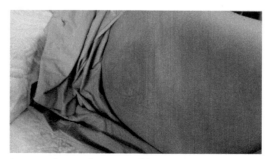

Fig. 8. Deep tissue damage. (*From* Shutterstock)

pain control, wound cleaning/debridement, infection prevention and treatment, wound dressing, topical treatments, and possible surgical interventions.[19,33,35]

When treating a patient with a pressure injury, it is important to assess pain control.[19] All patient's pain should be assessed regularly during treatment including psychological status.[19,38] Patients in the outpatient setting commonly have poorly controlled pain, which greatly affects their quality of life.[39] Nonpharmacologic treatments are first line, which include repositioning and support surfaces. If needed, patients should also have oral, intramuscular, or intravenous analgesics available particularly during dressing changes.[19]

Wound cleaning helps to remove dead tissue, decrease bacterial burden, and remove foreign bodies that can prevent tissue from healing.[19] Debridement also leads to faster healing time.[19,33] Cleaning solutions should be used if infection is suspected on the wound as well as surrounding skin. Hard eschars should be left in place unless there is a concern for infection.[19]

Assessing infections should be done regularly. Signs of infections include increased pain, warmth, erythema, and drainage or systemic systems.[19,33] Other signs of infection include delayed wound healing, wound breakdown/dehiscence, and necrotic tissue formation. Signs of a spreading infection include induration, crepitus of surrounding skin, lethargy, and systemic symptoms. Wounds should be evaluated for osteomyelitis if the bone is exposed.[19] Antibiotics should be used to treat infection covering for common skin flora as well as methicillin-resistant *Staphylococcus aureus*, pseudomonas, gram-negative rods, and anaerobes based on location of the wound and patient's comorbidities. Cultures should be collected particularly if there is an unexposed abscess or osteomyelitis to better direct antibiotic choices.[33] Evidence does not support the regular use of antiseptics on a wound without the presence of infection.[40]

Dressing selections should be based on the wound. Important considerations when selecting dressings are patient and/or care giver abilities, size and depth of injury, bacterial load, wound moisture, volume of exudate, condition of surrounding skin, presence of tunneling and/or undermining, and pain.[19] Dressings should be used to help maintain a good healing wound environment. Wet wounds should have dressings that remove extra moisture to prevent further breakdown in surrounding tissues, whereas dry wounds should use dressings that retain moisture to allow for better wound healing.[19,33] Negative pressure wound therapy can also be used to promote wound healing particularly in stages 3 and 4.[33]

Surgery may be warranted for certain populations with pressure injuries. Surgical evaluation should be done if there are concerns for a deep infection leading to sepsis, deep tissue not easily removed by conservative therapies, or wounds that are not closing with conservative therapies.[19] It is also important to assess if the patient is an appropriate candidate for surgery based on goals of care, clinical condition, and ability to complete treatment. Surgical debridement can be used to help clean wounds. Skin flaps and muscle flaps can also be used to close wounds, but there is a risk of dehiscence.[33,35] Patients with spinal cord injuries are at increased risk for recurrent pressure ulcers or dehiscence following flap closure.[35] Untreated infections also increase risk for dehiscence.[33] Partial removal of bony landmarks can also be considered to reduce boney prominence, thus decreasing risk for future pressure injuries.[33]

Wounds should be assessed regularly to ascertain if treatment regimens are working, usually on a weekly basis. It is important to make note of changes in size, characteristics of the wound bed itself, and surrounding tissue while monitoring for improvement.[19]

In addition to the medical complications of pressure injuries, pressure injuries also have significant physical, social, and psychological impact on quality of life.[24,38,39] These injuries commonly lead to decreased independence, social isolation, pain, fear, and anxiety.[24] A multimodal approach also aims at addressing these concerns when treating patients.

SUMMARY

Chronic wounds are commonly encountered in a family medicine practice. Identification of the type and the underlying, contributing conditions is important for management. Diagnostic imaging, laboratory evaluation, and tissue biopsy may be used to evaluate the wound. Surgical debridement or antibiotics have specific indications in the treatment of wounds. Consultation may be helpful in the management of underlying conditions.

CLINICS CARE POINTS

- Venous ulcers are the most common type of lower extremity ulcer. Diagnosis should always include venous duplex ultrasound as well as ankle brachial index to evaluate for arterial disease.

- The mainstay of treatment of venous ulcers is management of edema with compression; it also includes control of wound bed with combination of autolytic agents, surgical debridement, and antimicrobials if signs of bacterial infection are present.

- Intermittent compression devices may be a useful addition in the treatment of venous hypertension.

- Treatment of arterial ulcers must include addressing the underlying cause and will usually involve multiple specialties.

- The risk for pressure ulcers should be assessed using a validated scale in patients with limited mobility, poor nutrition, frailty, concomitant illness, or surgery. Avoidance of pressure, pressure relief devices, adequate nutrition, and addressing the wound are all required to prevent or treat pressure ulcers.

- Antibiotics are generally not needed for ulcers without increasing signs of infection or evidence of bone involvement in pressure ulcers.

DISCLOSURE

The authors have nothing to disclose.

SUPPLEMENTARY DATA

Supplementary data related to this article can be found online at 10.1016/j.pop.2021.10.009.

REFERENCES

1. Chung SL, Baruah M, Bahia SS. Diagnosis and management of venous leg ulcers. BMJ : Br Med J (Online) 2018;362. Available at: http://ezaccess.libraries.psu.edu/login?url=https://www-proquest-com.ezaccess.libraries.psu.edu/scholarly-journals/diagnosis-management-venous-leg-ulcers/docview/2088318557/se-2?accountid=13158. https://doi.org.ezaccess.libraries.psu.edu/10.1136/bmj.k3115.
2. Evangelista MT, Casintahan MF, Villafuerte LL. Simvastatin as a novel therapeutic agent for venous ulcers: a randomized, double-blind, placebo-controlled trial. Br J Dermatol 2014;170(5):1151–7.

3. Meissner MH, Moneta G, Burnand K, et al. The hemodynamics and diagnosis of venous disease. J Vasc Surg 2007;46(Suppl):S:4S–24S.

4. O'Donnell TF, Passman MA, Marston WA, et al. Management of venous leg ulcers: Clinical practice guidelines of the Society for Vascular Surgery® and the American Venous Forum. J Vasc Surg 2014;60(2). 3S-59S.

5. Rahim K, Saleha S, Zhu X, et al. Bacterial Contribution in Chronicity of Wounds. Microb Ecol 2017;73(3):710–21.

6. David R. Thomas, Managing Venous Stasis Disease and Ulcers. Clin Geriatr Med 2013;29(Issue 2):415–24.

7. Ubbink DT, Santema TB, Stoekenbroek RM. Systemic wound care: a meta-review of cochrane systematic reviews. Surg Technol Int 2014;24:99–111.

8. Fulbrook P, Mbuzi V, Miles S. Effectiveness of prophylactic sacral protective dressings to prevent pressure injury: A systematic review and meta-analysis. Int J Nurs Stud 2019;100:103400.

9. Gethin G, Cowman S, Kolbach DN. Debridement for venous leg ulcers. Cochrane Database Syst Rev 2015;2015(9):CD008599.

10. Briggs M, Nelson EA, Martyn-St James M. Topical agents or dressings for pain in venous leg ulcers. Cochrane Database Syst Rev 2012;11:CD001177. Accessed February 28, 2021.

11. O'Meara S, Cullum N, Nelson EA, et al. Compression for venous leg ulcers. Cochrane Database Syst Rev 2012;11(11):CD000265.

12. O'Meara S, Al-Kurdi D, Ologun Y, et al. Antibiotics and antiseptics for venous leg ulcers (Review). Cochrane Database Syst Rev 2014;(1):CD003557.

13. Gist S, Tio-Matos I, Falzgraf S, et al. Wound care in the geriatric client. Clin Interv Aging 2009;4:269–87.

14. Nelson EA, Hillman A, Thomas K. Intermittent pneumatic compression for treating venous leg ulcers. Cochrane Database Syst Rev 2014;5:CD001899.

15. Kirsner RS, Vivas AC. Lower extremity ulcers: diagnosis and management. Br J Dermatol 2015;173(2):379–90.

16. Fukaya E, Margolis D. Approach to diagnosing lower extremity ulcers. Dermol Ther May/june 2013;26(3):181–6.

17. Rozin AP, Egozi D, Ramon Y, et al. Large leg ulcers due to autoimmune diseases. Med Sci Monit 2011;17(1):CS1–7.

18. Edsberg LE, Black JM, Goldberg M, et al. Revised National Pressure Ulcer Advisory Panel Pressure Injury Staging System: Revised Pressure Injury Staging System. J Wound Ostomy Continence Nurs 2016;43(6):585–97.

19. National Pressure Ulcer Advisory Panel/European Pressure Ulcer Advisory Panel/ Pan Pacific Pressure Injury Alliance/(NPUAP/EPUAP/PPPIA). Prevention and treatment of pressure ulcers: quick reference guide can be found at NPUAP/ EPUAP/PPPIA 2019 PDF

20. Padula WV, Delarmente BA. The national cost of hospital-acquired pressure injuries in the United States. Int Wound J 2019;16(3):634–40.

21. Van Den Bos J, Rustagi K, Gray T, et al. The $17.1 billion problem: the annual cost of measurable medical errors. Health Aff (Millwood) 2011;30(4):596–603.

22. Russo CA, Steiner C, Spector W. Hospitalizations Related to Pressure Ulcers Among Adults 18 Years and Older, 2006: Statistical Brief #64. In: Healthcare cost and Utilization Project (HCUP) Statistical Briefs. Rockville (MD): Agency for Healthcare Research and Quality (US); 2006.

23. "Hospital-Acquired Condition Reduction Program." CMS.gov, US Centers for Medicare and Medicaid Services. Available at: https://www.cms.gov/Medicare/

Quality-Initiatives-Patient-Assessment-Instruments/Value-Based-Programs/HAC/Hospital-Acquired-Conditions. Accessed August 17 2021.

24. Mervis JS, Phillips TJ. Pressure ulcers: Pathophysiology, epidemiology, risk factors, and presentation. J Am Acad Dermatol 2019;81(4):881–90.

25. Vangilder C, Macfarlane GD, Meyer S. Results of nine international pressure ulcer prevalence surveys: 1989 to 2005. Ostomy Wound Manage 2008;54:40–54.

26. VanGilder C, Lachenbruch C, Algrim-Boyle C, et al. The International Pressure Ulcer Prevalence™ Survey: 2006-2015: A 10-Year Pressure Injury Prevalence and Demographic Trend Analysis by Care Setting. J Wound Ostomy Continence Nurs 2017;44(1):20–8.

27. Gefen A. The biomechanics of sitting-acquired pressure ulcers in patients with spinal cord injury or lesions. Int Wound J 2007;4(3):222–31.

28. Mimura M, Ohura T, Takahashi M, et al. Mechanism leading to the development of pressure ulcers based on shear force and pressures during a bed operation: influence of body types, body positions, and knee positions. Wound Repair Regen 2009;17(6):789–96.

29. Farage MA, Miller KW, Elsner P, et al. Characteristics of the aging skin. Adv Wound Care (New Rochelle) 2013;2:5–10.

30. Shaked E, Gefen A. Modeling the Effects of Moisture-Related Skin-Support Friction on the Risk for Superficial Pressure Ulcers during Patient Repositioning in Bed. Front Bioeng Biotechnol 2013;1:9.

31. Qaseem A, Mir TP, Starkey M, et al. Clinical Guidelines Committee of the American College of Physicians. Risk assessment and prevention of pressure ulcers: a clinical practice guideline from the American College of Physicians. Ann Intern Med 2015;162(5):359–69.

32. Lin F, Wu Z, Song B, et al. The effectiveness of multicomponent pressure injury prevention programs in adult intensive care patients: A systematic review. Int J Nurs Stud 2020;102:103483.

33. Mervis JS, Phillips TJ. Pressure ulcers: Prevention and management. J Am Acad Dermatol 2019;81(4):893–902.

34. Gillespie BM, Walker RM, Latimer SL, et al. Repositioning for pressure injury prevention in adults. Cochrane Database Syst Rev 2020;6(6):CD009958.

35. Qaseem A, Humphrey LL, Forciea MA, et al. Clinical Guidelines Committee of the American College of Physicians. Treatment of pressure ulcers: a clinical practice guideline from the American College of Physicians. Ann Intern Med 2015;162(5):370–9.

36. Munoz N, Posthauer ME, Cereda E, et al. The Role of Nutrition for Pressure Injury Prevention and Healing: The 2019 International Clinical Practice Guideline Recommendations. Adv Skin Wound Care 2020;33(3):123–36.

37. Lee SK, Posthauer ME, Dorner B, et al. Pressure ulcer healing with a concentrated, fortified, collagen protein hydrolysate supplement: a randomized controlled trial. Adv Skin Wound Care 2006;19(2):92–6.

38. Kim J, Lyon D, Weaver MT, et al. Demographics, Psychological Distress, and Pain From Pressure Injury. Nurs Res 2019;68(5):339–47.

39. Jackson D, Durrant L, Bishop E, et al. Pain associated with pressure injury: A qualitative study of community-based, home-dwelling individuals. J Adv Nurs 2017;73(12):3061–9.

40. Norman G, Dumville JC, Moore ZE, et al. Antibiotics and antiseptics for pressure ulcers. Cochrane Database Syst Rev 2016;4(4):CD011586.

Dermoscopy in Primary Care

Prabhat K. Pokhrel, MS, MD, PhD, FAAFP[a],*, Matthew F. Helm, MD[b],
Amrit Greene, MD[b], Leesha A. Helm, MD, MPH[c], Michael Partin, MD[c]

KEYWORDS

- Dermoscopy • Melanocytic • Nonmelanocytic • Nevi • Dermatofibroma
- Seborrheic keratosis • Melanoma • Carcinoma

KEY POINTS

- Dermoscopy increases diagnostic accuracy and sensitivity for detecting melanoma.
- Introduce commonly used algorithms in basic dermoscopy.
- Specific findings for basal cell and squamous cell carcinoma aid the examiner in making decisions on when to biopsy.
- Introduce resources to the primary care providers to improve diagnostic skills in dermoscopy.

INTRODUCTION TO DERMATOSCOPE AND DERMOSCOPY

The incidence of skin cancer in the United States is greater than the incidence of all other cancers combined. The incidence of basal cell carcinoma (BCC), squamous cell carcinoma (SCC), and melanoma are all on the rise.[1] The aim of this article is to introduce primary care providers (PCPs) to specific and characteristic dermoscopic features of benign and malignant lesions, and to help develop a basic framework and algorithm to assist in deciding whether a lesion needs to be biopsied.

Dermoscopy is a noninvasive technique that allows in vivo magnification (x 10–20) of the skin structures and helps in visualizing microscopic features that are imperceptible to the naked eye. Dermoscopy is not a substitute for biopsy and histopathologic evaluation, but is an important tool that can help increase diagnostic sensitivity and specificity of cutaneous lesions.

A dermatoscope is a small and portable handheld device with a polarized and a nonpolarized mode that permits toggling between more superficial and deeper structures. Polarized and nonpolarized modes are complementary to each other and provide additional information. Visit https://dermlitestore.com/products/dermlite-dl4 for more information on dermatoscopes.

[a] Family Medicine Residency, Department of Family Medicine, McLaren Flint, G-3230 Beecher Road, Ste 1, Flint, MI 48532, USA; [b] Department of Dermatology, Penn State Hersey Medical Center, 500 University Drive, Hersey, PA 17033, USA; [c] Department of Family and Community Medicine, Penn State Hersey Medical Center, 500 University Drive, Hersey, PA 17033, USA
* Corresponding author.
E-mail address: prabhat.pokhrel@mclaren.org

Prim Care Clin Office Pract 49 (2022) 99–118
https://doi.org/10.1016/j.pop.2021.10.004
0095-4543/22/© 2021 Elsevier Inc. All rights reserved.

A nonpolarized dermatoscope (NPD) helps better visualize the superficial color and structures of the cutaneous lesions. Light reflected by the stratum corneum can be reduced by using ultrasound gel or alcohol to better visualize the structures. Polarized dermoscopy (PD) does not require a liquid interface or direct skin contact. Ability of PD to see vascular structures depends on the pressure applied by the dermatoscope to the lesion. PD allows for better penetration and appreciation of deeper structures such as vasculature and collagen.[2]

Dermoscopy increases the diagnostic sensitivity compared with naked eye examination (NEE).[3] Diagnostic sensitivity of melanoma with NEE is only 38%, whereas with dermoscopy it is about 72%.[4] Dermoscopy decreases the number of biopsies needed to find a skin cancer from 12 to 18:1 to 4 to 5:1.[5,6] A significant improvement in diagnostic accuracy for benign and malignant lesions has been reported among family medicine physicians after an introductory training course on dermoscopy.[7]

DERMOSCOPIC TERMINOLOGIES, COLORS, AND STRUCTURES

Familiarity with key terms, common colors, and structures used in dermoscopy is essential and helps health care providers decide whether biopsy is warranted. Skin layers combine to produce important colors and patterns that are crucial dermoscopic features. Colors and structures specific to benign melanocytic lesions, melanoma, and their odds ratio for melanoma are outlined in **Table 1**.

The most relevant colors when evaluating cutaneous neoplasms with dermoscopy are black, brown, blue, gray, yellow, orange, red, and white. Most of these colors are attributed to increased amounts melanin (brown, black, gray, blue), blood (red), sebum or keratin (yellow), or collagen (white).[8] Melanin is the most common chromophore, and the color of the skin will vary from black to brown to blue-gray depending on its concentration and location (**Figure 1**, **Table 2**). Colors can provide valuable insight into the depth of a melanocytic lesion.[8,9]

COLORS AND STRUCTURES OF MELANOCYTIC LESIONS

Dermoscopy is useful in the evaluation of pigmented lesions. Dermoscopic structures that are specific for melanocytic skin lesions are pigment network, negative network, angulated lines, dot, and globules (**Figs. 2–4**).[8] Melanocytic lesions can either be benign or malignant.

Benign Patterns of Melanocytic Lesions

A benign lesion generally has uniform pattern, homogeneous pigment distribution and is symmetric. Examples of benign melanocytic lesions are common acquired nevus, Spitz nevus, blue nevus and congenital nevus.

Common acquired nevus (mole)

Clinically, an acquired nevus appears as a flat to elevated pigmented lesion mainly on the sun-exposed areas of the skin. The borders are usually regular and well-defined. Common dermoscopic patterns of acquired melanocytic nevi are reticular, globular, cobblestone, reticulo-globular, and homogeneous. Each of these patterns may manifest typical/atypical network, small/large globules, symmetric streaks, and regular/irregular dots.[10] Growing nevi often reveal a peripheral rim of small homogenous, brown globules. It is not uncommon to have central hyper or hypopigmentation in acquired nevus (see **Fig. 3**). Many of these patterns can be seen in benign nevi and melanoma. Therefore, it is important to consider the lesion en mass to identify uniformity (benign) or asymmetry with multiple patterns that increase suspicion of malignancy.

Table 1

Dermoscopic melanoma-specific structures, and their odds ratios for melanoma

Metaphorical Terms	Description	Odds Ratio For Melanoma
Atypical pigment network and angulated lines	Network with increased variability in the color, thickness, distribution, or spacing of the lines; when angulated, typically they show gray color	2–9
Negative pigment network	Serpiginous interconnecting broadened hypopigmented lines that surround elongated and curvilinear globules	1.4–1.8
Irregular dots/globules	Clods with variability in color, size, shape, or spacing and distributed in an asymmetric fashion	1.7–4.8
Irregular streaks (pseudopods, radial streaming)	Radial lines with bulbous projections (pseudopods) or without (radial streaming) irregularly distributed	1.5–5.8
Granularity/peppering and scarlike depigmentation	Granularity: blue-gray dots; scarlike depigmentation: white area lighter than surrounding skin devoid of vessels and shiny white structures	2–18.3
Blue-whitish veil	Homogenous blue white area overlying a raised area	1.74–13
Shiny white streaks	Short white lines oriented parallel and orthogonal to each other (only see with PD)	2.5–9.7
Irregular blotch	Off-centered blotch or multiple blotches	1.88–4.1
Polymorphous vessels	Simultaneous presence of multiple types of vessels	2.0–3.04

Adapted from Braun R. Vascular structures. Dermoscopedia. June 17, 2019, 09:29 UTC. Available at: https://dermoscopedia.org/w/index.php?title=Vascular_structures&oldid=16709. Accessed December 21, 2020. From Dermoscopedia with permission.

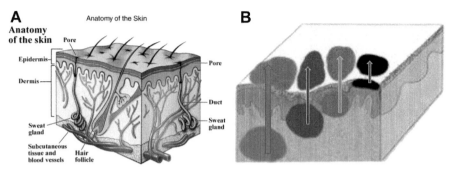

Fig. 1. (*A*) Anatomy of skin. (*B*) Relationship between depth of melanin and color visualization through dermoscope. (*Adapted from* Oriol Yélamos, Katrin Kerl, Ralph Braun, Daniel Morgado, Constanza Riquelme Mc Loughlin. Colors. Dermoscopedia. February 6, 2020, 10:15 UTC. Available at: https://dermoscopedia.org/w/index.php?title=Colors&oldid=17064. Accessed December 21, 2020. From Dermscopedia with permission.)

Spitz/reed nevus

Clinically, Spitz nevi (SN) are well-circumscribed, dome-shaped papules or nodules that vary in color (pink, tan, dark brown, or black) and in size (2 mm to >2 cm). They are generally homogenous in color with well-defined margins. They can occur in any age group but most patients are under 20 years of age, and nevi usually occur on the lower extremities, head, and neck area. Reed nevus (RN) is a benign lesion, usually flat or slightly raised, dark brown to black with a well-defined border.

Argenziano and colleagues described the dermoscopic aspects of pigmented SN and correlated them to specific histopathologic features. The 3 main dermoscopic patterns of PSN are (1) a globular pattern (22%, **Fig. 5**A), (2) a starburst pattern (53%, **Fig. 5**B), and (3) an atypical pattern (25%, **Fig. 5**C, D).[11] The starburst pattern is characterized by prominent, black to blue diffuse pigmentation and pseudopods distributed regularly at the periphery in a radiate pattern. The globular pattern is typified by a discrete, brown to gray-blue pigmentation and a peripheral rim of large brown globules often extending throughout the entire lesion. At its early stage, an SN may have more of a globular appearance followed by the starburst pattern. These patterns should be considered as different morphologic expressions corresponding to the evolutionary phases of pigmented SN (see **Fig. 5**).[12]

Clinically, histopathologically, and dermoscopically, SN and RN may mimic melanoma, or melanoma may mimic SN (spitzoid melanoma). Nevertheless, dermoscopy helps to enhance diagnostic accuracy from 46% to 93%.[13]

Table 2 Color of melanin under dermatoscope based on location	
Skin Layer	**Color**
Stratum corneum	Black
Dermo-epidermal junction (DEJ)	Brown
Papillary dermis	Gray
Reticular dermis	Blue

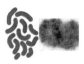 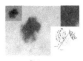 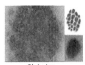

| Pigment Network | Negative network | Angulated lines | Dots | Globules |

Fig. 2. Dermoscopic structures that are specific for melanocytic skin lesions. (*Adapted from* Oriol Yélamos, Katrin Kerl, Ralph Braun. Pigment network. Dermoscopedia. February 6, 2020, 10:36 UTC. Available at: https://dermoscopedia.org/w/index.php?title=Pigment_ network&oldid=17071. Accessed December 21, 2020. From Dermoscopedia with permission.)

Congenital melanocytic nevus

Clinically, congenital melanocytic nevi (CMNs) are brown, oval, and symmetric lesions. They can be raised and have a cobblestone texture, with or without hypertrichosis.

In adults, CMNs are classified by their size: small (<1.5 cm in diameter), medium (1.5–20 cm), large (>20–40 cm), and giant (>40 cm at their greatest diameter). Although smaller CMNs rarely transform into melanoma, about 2% of large/giant CMNs transform into melanoma.[14] Therefore, patients with large/giant CMNs should be instructed to monitor their CMNs for change.

There are no specific dermoscopic criteria for CMNs, so dermoscopy can be used to support a clinical diagnosis.[15] Dermoscopic patterns of CMN vary according to age and location. The most common patterns in CMN are reticular, globular, and reticulo-globular (see **Figs. 3** and **4**). Hypertrichosis, blood vessels, and pigmentary changes may also be seen in CMNs. Globular patterns are much more common in those who are younger than 12 years while a reticular pattern is observed exclusively in individuals aged 12 years or older. Globular patterns are more common in the head, neck, and extremities, while a reticular pattern is more common in the extremities.[16]

Blue nevus

Clinically, the common blue nevus is characterized by dark blue/black macules usually between 5 and 10 mm in diameter. They can occur anywhere but about 50% are on the dorsal aspect of the hands and face. They are blue tumors of dermal melanocytes, and thus the pigment is deeper than in ordinary nevi. Because of their dark color, they can raise suspicion for melanoma.

Dermoscopically, the common blue nevus shows a homogenous structure-less blue, blue-gray to blue-black pattern with a symmetric border (**Fig. 6**A). They often lack pigment network, but peripheral regular streaks have been described

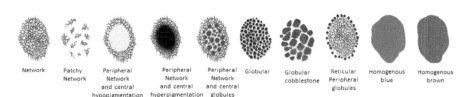

| Network | Patchy Network | Peripheral Network and central hypopigmentation | Peripheral Network and central hyperpigmentation | Peripheral Network and central globules | Globular | Globular cobblestone | Reticular Peripheral globules | Homogenous blue | Homogenous brown |

Fig. 3. The most common patterns found in nevi. (*Adapted from* Ralph Braun, Aimilios Lallas, Ash Marghoob. Level 1: Nevi. Dermoscopedia. September 10, 2018, 21:39 UTC. Available at: https://dermoscopedia.org/w/index.php?title=Level_1:_Nevi&oldid=13536. Accessed October 16, 2020. From Dermoscopedia with permission.)

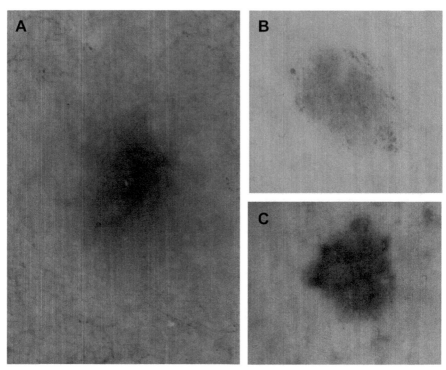

Fig. 4. Melanocytic nevi under dermoscopy. (*A*) Compound dysplastic nevus congenital type. (*B*) Melanocytic nevus with comma shaped vessels. (*C*) Melanocytc nevus with reticulated pattern. (*Courtesy of* Amrit Greene, MD, Hershey, PA)

(**Fig. 6**B).[17] Irregular streaks in a similar lesion could be melanoma (**Fig. 6**C). There may be white areas caused by fibrosis, and the pigment in blue nevi are usually confluent and fade toward the periphery. When evaluating these lesions, it is important to check for the absence of additional dermoscopic features such as atypical vessels, streaks, dots/globules, and network, which is crucial in distinguishing from other melanocytic lesions such as melanoma.[18]

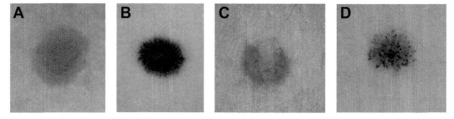

Fig. 5. Reed-Spitz nevi at different evolutionary phases. (*A*) Globular pattern. (*B*) Starburst pattern. (*C* and *D*) Atypical pattern. (*Adapted from* Michael Kunz, Ralph Braun. Evolution of Spitz nevi. Dermoscopedia. June 28, 2017, 06:06 UTC. Available at: https://dermoscopedia. org/w/index.php?title=Evolution_of_Spitz_nevi&oldid=5207. Accessed October 16, 2020. From Dermoscopedia with permission.)

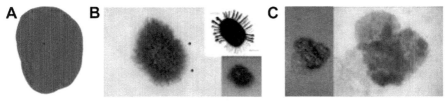

Fig. 6. (*A*) Homogeneous blue pattern (blue nevus). (*B*) Regular streaks (blue Nevus). (*C*) Irregular streaks/psudopods (melanoma). (*Adapted from* [A] Ralph Braun, Oriol Yélamos. Homogenous blue pattern. Dermoscopedia. May 20, 2019, 12:45 UTC. Available at: https://dermoscopedia.org/w/index.php?title=Homogenous_blue_pattern&oldid=15805. Accessed February 22, 2021. From Dermoscopedia with permission; and [B,C] Ralph Braun. Irregular Streaks. Dermoscopedia. July 8, 2018, 10:44 UTC. Available at: https://dermoscopedia.org/w/index.php?title=Irregular_Streaks&oldid=12446. Accessed February 22, 2021. From Dermoscopedia with permission.)

Melanoma-Specific Patterns

The commonly used ABCDE rule (asymmetry, border, color, diameter, and evolution) for clinical diagnosis of melanoma is unreliable and does not help to distinguish between pigmented and nonpigmented lesions.

Use of dermoscopy has been shown to significantly improve the diagnosis of melanocytic lesions. Algorithms used in diagnosing melanoma should include pattern analysis (triage amalgamated dermoscopic algorithm [TADA] or 2-xtep), the ABCD rule, the Menzis method, or the 7-point checklist, revised or classic. Argenziano and colleagues described in detail the classic and revised 7-point checklist. In summary, a lesion with a score of at least 3 with the classic tool, and score of at least 1 should be biopsied when the revised 7-point checklist is used.[19]

Dermoscopic characteristics that are associated with cutaneous melanoma are shown in **Figs. 7** and **8** and **Table 1**. Histopathologic correlates of dermoscopic features are outlined in **Table 3**.[20]

Some dermoscopic characteristics that indicate the presence of invasive melanomas include the presence of 2 or more colors, ulceration, no pigmentation, pseudopods, or f blue white veil. Other common characteristics include changes in the distribution pattern of color characterized by the combination of 2 or more colors or

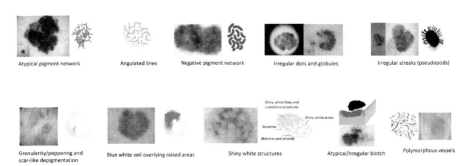

Fig. 7. Dermoscopic structures that are specific for melanoma. (*Adapted from* Ralph Braun, Katrin Kerl. Dermoscopic structures. Dermoscopedia. June 9, 2019, 12:38 UTC. Available at: https://dermoscopedia.org/w/index.php?title=Dermoscopic_structures&oldid=16549. Accessed February 22, 2021. From Dermoscopedia with permission.)

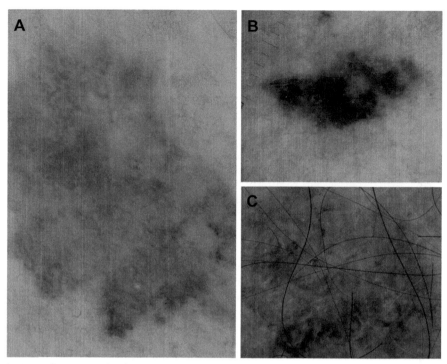

Fig. 8. Melanoma under dermatoscope. (*A*) Note the asymmetry, irregular borders, negative network and irregular pigment network. (*B*) Note the obstruction of follicular ostia, off-center blotch, and atypical pigment network. (*C*) Note the asymmetry, negative network, asymmetric perifollicular pigment, and shiny white lines. (*Courtesy of* Amrit Greene, MD, Hershey, PA)

by the presence of irregular pigmented dots.[21] Melanomas in acral surfaces, face, mucosa, and nail have different patterns and will not be discussed here.

Amelanotic melanomas are rare but difficult to diagnose, although dermoscopy has improved accuracy. The most positive predictors of amelanotic and hypomelanotic melanoma are, in order, having a blue-white veil, scarlike depigmentation, multiple blue-gray dots, irregularly shaped depigmentation, brown dots or globules irregular in size or distribution, 5 to 6 colors, predominant central vessels, red-blue color, and peripheral light brown structure-less areas greater than 10% of the lesion.[22]

Nonmelanocytic Lesions

Commonly encountered nonmelanocytic lesions include BCC, SCC, dermatofibroma, seborrheic keratosis (SK), cherry angioma, solar lentigo, and sebaceous hyperplasia. Only the first 5 lesions will be discussed here.

Basal cell carcinoma

Lesions in BCC are slow growing with rare metastasis, but can lead to significant morbidity through local tissue destruction.[18,23] Clinically, BCC can manifest with different morphologies from patch to plaques to nodules and may mimic melanoma.[18] Two common subtypes of BCC are nodular and superficial.[23,24] Nodular BCC, accounts for approximately 80% of cases, generally affects the face and has the

Table 3
Dermoscopy-histopathologic relationship

Dermoscopic Feature	Histopathologic Correlate
Typical pigment network	Pigmented and elongated rete ridges with increased number of melanocytes
Black dots	Focal collections of melanocytes and clumps of melanin within the stratum corneum
Brown globules	Discrete junctional nests of more or less pigmented melanocytes or nevus cells in the papillary dermis.
Blue-white veil	Acanthotic epidermis with compact orthokeratosis with more or less pronounced hypergranulosis usually overlying a large melanin-containing area in the dermis
Hypopigmentation	Decrease in melanin pigmentation in the epidermis or dermis
Milialike cysts	Intraepidermal horn globules (horn psudocysts)
Comedolike openings	Keratin plugs within dilated follicular openings
Leaflike areas	Pigmented solid aggregations of basaloid cells in the papillary dermis
White areas	Fibrosis within a more or less thickened papillary dermis

From Massi D, De Giorgi V, Soyer HP. Histopathologic correlates of dermoscopic criteria. Dermatol Clin 2001;19(2):259-68, vii.

appearance of a pearly papule with telangiectases.[23,25] Superficial BCCs are typically thin plaques or scaly patches characterized by central clearing commonly located on the trunk. Typically, BCC does not invade subcutaneous tissue.

BCCs dermoscopically portray classic characteristic features such as arborizing blood vessels translucency (**Figs. 9–12**)

Spoke wheel-like structures enclosing a central hyperpigmented area that is blue-gray in color (see **Figs. 9**B and **11**)

Brown or blue-gray leaflike structures (see **Fig. 9**C)

Multiple blue-gray ovoid nests and/or globules in a random pattern (see **Fig. 9**D,E and **11**)

Shiny white patches

Blotches and linear strands (see **Figs. 9**F and **11**) that can only be seen with PD

Ulceration (see **Fig. 9**G)[8,18,23,26]

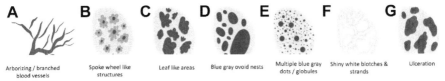

Fig. 9. Features associated with BCC. (*A*) Arborizing / branched blood vessels. (*B*) Spoke wheel like structures. (*C*) Leaf like areas. (*D*) Blue gray ovoid nests. (*E*) Multiple blue gray dots/ globules. (*F*) Shiny white blotches & strands. (*G*) Ulceration. (*Adapted from* Ash Marghoob, Natalia Jaimes. Basal cell carcinoma. Dermoscopedia. June 8, 2019, 11:10 UTC. Available at: https://dermoscopedia.org/w/index.php?title=Basal_cell_carcinoma&oldid=16531. Accessed February 22, 2021. From Dermoscopedia with permission.)

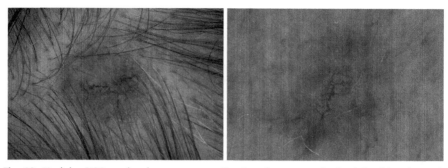

Fig. 10. Nodular BCCs under dermoscopy; notice translucency and arborizing blood vessels. (*Courtesy of* Amrit Greene, MD, Hershey, PA)

Arborizing vessels (see **Fig. 10**), blue gray ovoid nest, and ulceration are specific for nodular BCC, while spoke wheel, fine telangiectasias and leaflike structures are indicative of superficial BCC.[27]

Squamous cell carcinoma

SCC is the second most common primary nonmelanotic skin cancer, accounting for approximately 20% of cases.[27]

Dermatoscopic structures of keratinizing tumors like SCC, actinic keratosis (AK), and Bowen disease (BD) depend on subtypes. Dermoscopic features of AKs include strawberry pattern of erythema surrounding a hair follicle that is red-pink, superficial

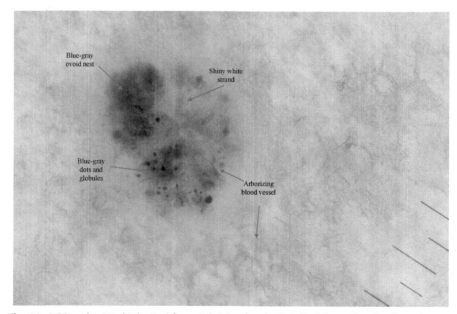

Fig. 11. BCC under PD. (*Adapted from* Ash Marghoob, Natalia Jaimes. Basal cell carcinoma. Dermoscopedia. June 8, 2019, 11:10 UTC. Available at: https://dermoscopedia.org/w/index. php?title=Basal_cell_carcinoma&oldid=16531. Accessed September 16, 2020. From Dermoscopedia with permission.)

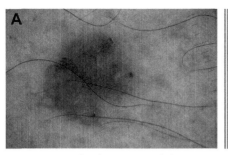 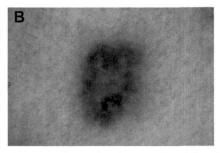

Fig. 12. BCC under dermoscopy. (*A*) Notice central erosion, shiny white lines, and peripheral blue gray ovoid nest. (*B*) Notice blue/gray ovoid nests and leaflike structures at periphery. (*Courtesy of* Amrit Greene, MD, Hershey, PA.)

yellow scale, wavy blood vessels around the follicle (**Fig. 13**), and nonspecific white 4-leaf clover-shaped lesion known as rosette sign (see **Fig. 13**A; **Fig. 14**).[28,29] Dermoscopic criteria for BD are coiled (glomerular) vessels, pink or skin-colored structureless areas and disorganized brown or gray dots in linear arrangement, scaly surface, focal, asymmetric distribution of vessels (**Fig. 15**).[27,30]

Well-differentiated SCC is characterized dermoscopically by a collection of central brown-yellow keratin, scales with uniform looped, pinpoint, or serpentine vessels (**Fig. 16**).[18,26] Poorly differential SCC demonstrates ulceration, bleeding, and diffuse arrangements of blood vessels covering more than 50% of the tumor surface.[27,31]

Dermatofibroma

Dermatofibroma is a common slow-growing benign tumor that may occur in any age group. It mostly affects young and middle-aged adults, with a 2:1 female-to-male predominance. Clinically, it is a 1 cm or less in diameter, solitary or multiple, firm nontender papule(s), plaque(s), or nodule(s) with a smooth surface. Its color may range from light to dark brown, purple to red or yellow. The dimple sign created after lateral compression of opposite side of the lesion is a characteristic sign of dermatofibroma. They are commonly found on the lower extremities. Patients often relate dermatofibroma to a minor skin injury.[32] The most common dermatoscopic pattern of dermatofibroma is central white patch and peripheral pigment network that may be seen in up

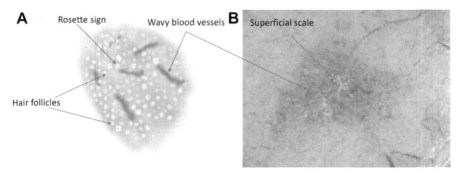

Fig. 13. Actinic keratosis with strawberry pattern. (*A*) Rosette sign, wavy blood vessels, hair follicles. (*B*) Wavy blood vessels and superficial scale. (*From* Ralph Braun. Strawberry pattern. Dermoscopedia. May 24, 2019, 15:34 UTC. Available at: https://dermoscopedia.org/w/index.php?title=Strawberry_pattern&oldid=16190. Accessed September 16, 2020. From Dermoscopedia with permission.)

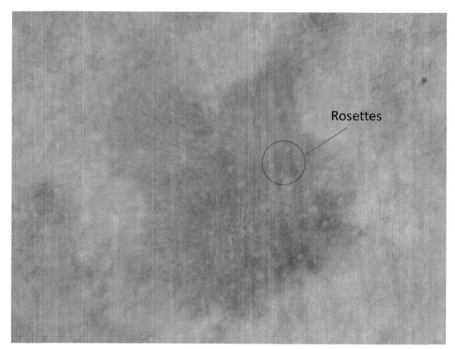

Fig. 14. Rosettes. (*Adapted from* Ralph Braun. Rosettes. Dermoscopedia. May 21, 2019, 09:29 UTC. Available at: https://dermoscopedia.org/w/index.php?title=Rosettes&oldid=15859. Accessed September 16, 2020. From Dermoscopedia with permission.)

to 35% of patients with dermatofibroma. Other dermatoscopic features of dermatofibroma could be delicate pigment network throughout, peripheral delicate pigment network and central white network, white network throughout, and absence of melanocytic features (**Fig. 17**).[33]

Seborrheic keratosis

SK is a common benign skin lesion with a prevalence of 50% to 80% in adults over 50 years of age. It is a nonmalignant epithelial neoplasm with a wide range of clinical and dermoscopic features. Most often SKs can be diagnosed clinically with an unaided eye because of their size (few millimeters to centimeters), color (light to dark brown), and stuck on symmetric appearance, which could be waxy plaques, papules or nodules. Dermoscopic features seen commonly with SK can help clinicians in making the accurate diagnosis. Some uncommon SK lesions, such as deeply pigmented SK, may lack typical dermoscopic features and could mimic malignant skin lesions.[34] Irritated SK (ISK), which is a unique variant of SK, and SCC, may have significant dermoscopic similarities, while other features are more characteristics either of ISK or SCC. For example, dotted or branched linear blood vessels, peripheral arrangement of vessels, and white structureless areas are more common dermoscopic features of SCC.[35]

Most SKs manifest typical dermoscopic features that increase the clinical diagnostic accuracy of SK and help avoid unnecessary biopsy. Dermoscopy, as a complementary tool to the history and physical examination, is the preferred nonsurgical diagnostic tool to differentiate pigmented SK from other pigmented tumors like

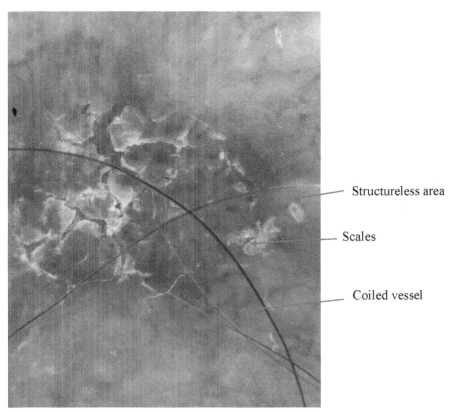

Structureless area

Scales

Coiled vessel

Fig. 15. Bowen disease with glomerular vessels and scales. (*Adapted from* Florentia Dimitriou, Theresa Deinlein, Iris Zalaudek. Bowen's disease. Dermoscopedia. June 8, 2019, 11:23 UTC. Available at: https://dermoscopedia.org/w/index.php?title=Bowen%27s_disease&oldid=16542. Accessed September 16, 2020. From Dermoscopedia with permission.)

cutaneous melanoma.[36,37] If the diagnosis of SK or its variants is questionable, or if the lesion is severely irritated, inflamed, ulcerated, crusted, bleeding, or rapidly changing, biopsy of the lesion should be performed for histopathological confirmation.

Dermoscopic criteria of SK are: multiple milialike cysts, comedolike openings, fissures/ridges, fat fingers, hairpin vessels, moth-eaten border, opaque-brown pigmentation, micalike structure, yellowish color, sharp demarcation, focal hemorrhage, grapelike vessels, coral-like structure, globulelike structure, and networklike structures (**Figs. 18 and 19**).[38]

Milialike cysts (see **Fig. 18**A, B) are white to yellow round structures that are visible in pigmented and nonpigmented SK. They are seen better under NPD than under PD (**Fig. 20**). They can also be found in BCC, congenital nevi and melanoma. Therefore, they are not pathognomonic for SK. If BCC is excluded, 3 or more milialike cysts in nonmelanocytic lesions are diagnostic of SK unless proven otherwise.[39]

Comedolike openings (see **Fig. 18**A, B) are brownish holes and correspond to keratin-filled invaginations on the surface of the epidermis. They are also known as crypts.[39]

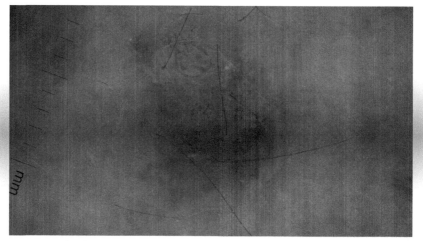

Fig. 16. SCC under dermoscopy. Note the glomeruloid vessels, white circles and scale. (*Courtesy of* Amrit Greene, MD, Hershey, PA)

Fissures and ridges (see **Fig. 18**A, C) give SK the appearance of brain surface (gyri and sulci) and has a cerebriform look.[39]

Fingerprints (see **Fig. 18**A, D) are small gyri and look like fingerprints. They are longer and wider in appearance.[39]

Cherry angioma

Clinically, cherry angioma is a nontender, smooth, dome-shaped, firm bright papule ranging between 0.5 and 5 mm in diameter. It is the most common acquired vascular lesion in adults and increases with age (75% in adults over 75 years of age). It tends to occur more often on the trunk or upper extremities, often multiple in numbers but asymptomatic, except bleeding with trauma. Unless fibrotic, cherry angioma blanches with applied pressure. Cherry angioma does not turn into malignant lesions, but may resemble amelanotic melanoma.[40] Dermoscopically, cherry angiomas are

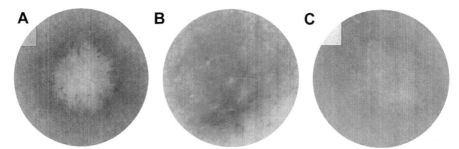

Fig. 17. Dermoscopic features of Dermatofibroma: (*A*) Peripheral delicate pigment network and central white scar-like patch, (*B*) Delicate pigment network throughout, (*C*) White network throughout. (*Adapted from* Ignacio Gómez Martín, Pedro Zaballos. Dermatofibromas. Dermoscopedia. June 3, 2019, 06:19 UTC. Available at: https://dermoscopedia.org/w/index.php?title=Dermatofibromas&oldid=16373. Accessed December 9, 2020. From Dermoscopedia with permission.)

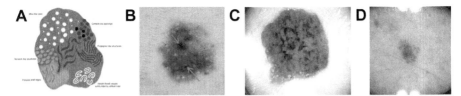

Fig. 18. (*A*) Schematics of milialike cysts, comedolike openings, fissure and ridges and finger like structures. (*B*) Milialike cysts under dermatoscope (red *arrows*) and comedolike openings (*blue arrows*) (*C*) Fissure and ridges under dermoscope. (*D*) Fingerlike structures under dermatoscope. (*Adapted from* Ralph Braun, Stephanie Nouveau, Sabine Ludwig. Seborrheic keratoses. Dermoscopedia. June 6, 2019, 16:40 UTC. Available at: https://dermoscopedia.org/w/index.php?title=Seborrheic_keratoses&oldid=16505. Accessed December 23, 2020. From Dermoscopedia with permission.)

amelanocytic with well-circumscribed lagoons (lacunae) of red or reddish maroon-coloring (**Fig. 21**). If capillaries are thrombosed, color may change from red to blue or black.

DERMOSCOPIC ALGORITHM
Triage Amalgamated Dermoscopic Algorithm

TADA is a step-wise, easy-to-use algorithm designed to help primary care providers in deciding whether to biopsy a lesion or not.[41,42] It is one of the few widely used triage algorithms. Further management strategy is based on clinical and dermoscopic characteristics of the lesion being investigated. Sensitivity and specificity of TADA for all skin cancers have been reported to be 88.1% to 94.6% (95% confidence interval [CI] = 93.4-95.7%) and 72.5% to 87.8% (95% CI = 70.1-74.7%), respectively.[41] After attending a 1-day course on dermoscopy, a significant improvement physicians' ability to diagnose dermatofibromas, angiomas, and seborrheic keratoses using TADA was observed.[42] In step 1 of TADA, the goal is to make sure the lesion is unequivocally SK, cherry angioma, or DF. Diagnosis of SK and DF may require visualization under PD and NPD lights. If the lesion is one of these 3 lesions, counseling, reassuring, and self-monitoring with a periodic follow-up is appropriate. If the lesion is not SK, cherry angioma, or DF, then steps 2 and 3 of TADA are followed using polarized light. In step 2, attention is paid to the pattern of distribution of colors or structures (organized vs disorganized patter). A lesion with a disorganized pattern needs to undergo a bi opsy, or the patient needs to be referred to a dermatologist for further evaluation of

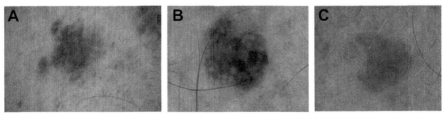

Fig. 19. SK . (*A*) Fingerlike structures under dermatoscope. (*B*) Milialike cysts under dermatoscope and comedolike openings. (*C*) Fissure and ridges under dermatoscope. (*Courtesy of* Amrit Greene, MD, Hershey, PA)

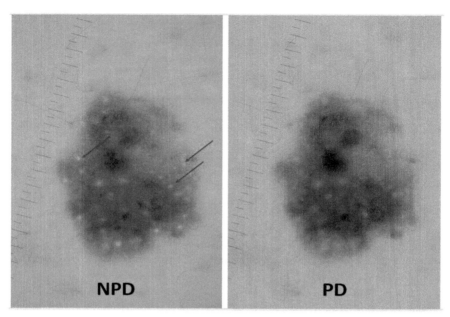

Fig. 20. Milialike cysts (*red arrows*) seen better under NPD compared with PD. (*Adapted from* Alon Scope. Principles of dermoscopy. Dermoscopedia. February 2, 2020, 11:39 UTC. Available at: https://dermoscopedia.org/w/index.php?title=Principles_of_dermoscopy&oldid=17040. Accessed December 23, 2020. From Dermoscopedia with permission.)

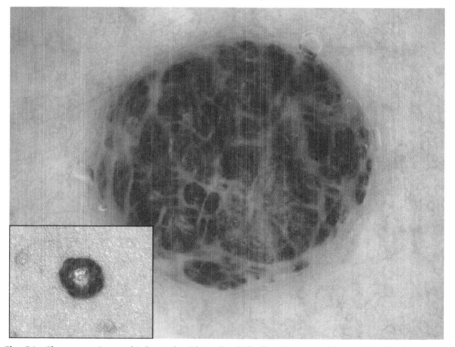

Fig. 21. Cherry angioma. (*Adapted with* Pedro Zaballos, Ignacio Gómez Martín. Angioma. Dermoscopedia. December 28, 2018, 17:10 UTC. Available at: https://dermoscopedia.org/w/index.php?title=Angioma&oldid=14607. Accessed December 10, 2020. From Dermoscopedia with permission.)

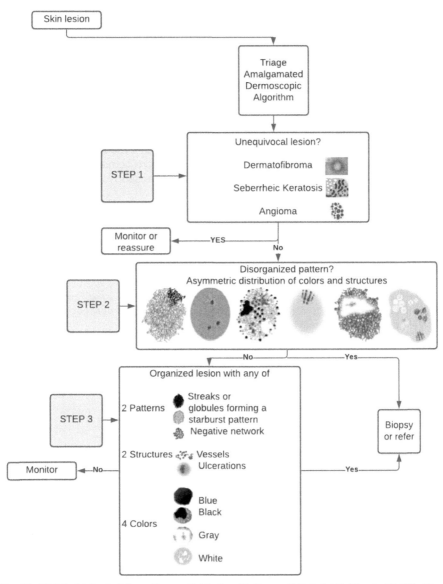

Fig. 22. TADA. (*Adapted from* Rogers T, Marino M, Dusza SW, Bajaj S, Marchetti MA, Marghoob A. Triage amalgamated dermoscopic algorithm (TADA) for skin cancer screening. Dermatol Pract Concept. 2017;7(2):9. DOI: https://doi.org/10.5826/dpc.0702a09; with permission.)

the lesion. If a lesion manifests an organized pattern of distribution of its color and structures, step 3 of TADA is followed through. In step 3, providers should pay attention to 2 patterns (starburst pattern formed from streaks or globules and negative network), 2 structures (vessels or ulceration without trauma), and 4 colors (blue, black, gray or white). White color may include shiny structures, circles, and scar-like areas). If step 3 reveals any of the previously mentioned patterns, structures, or colors, the lesion must undergo biopsy or the patient must be referred appropriately. Lesions without any of these patterns, structures, or colors may be monitored (**Fig. 22**).[41]

SUMMARY

PCPs are often the first line in encountering and managing skin lesions, including skin cancers. However, lack of training in the detection and management of skin cancers may lead to its mismanagement. It has been demonstrated that even a short course on dermoscopy can improve PCPs' abilities to identify malignant versus nonmalignant lesions and decide which lesions are appropriate for biopsy.[4,42] This article provided an introduction to dermoscopic features in order to help PCPs recognize concerning lesions and help classify common skin growths. For a more comprehensive overview, the authors recommend reading An Atlas of Dermoscopy by Marghoob and colleagues.[43]

CLINICS CARE POINTS

- Dermoscopy is a helpful adjunct for analyzing skin lesions, but it is not to replace clinical suspicion.
- The first step in evaluating a lesion is to determine whether it has a melanocytic network, then determine if it falls nicely into a common benign pattern; if it does not, consider biopsying to rule out melanoma
- Learning lesion-specific structures will help the clinician to more accurately determine what a lesion is and whether it deserves a biopsy.

DISCLOSURE

The authors have nothing to disclose.

REFERENCES

1. Rigel DS, Friedman RJ, Kopf AW. Lifetime risk for development of skin cancer in the U.S. population: current estimate is now 1 in 5. J Am Acad Dermatol 1996; 35(6):1012–3.
2. Pan Y, Gareau DS, Scope A, et al. Polarized and nonpolarized dermoscopy: the explanation for the observed differences. Arch Dermatol 2008;144(6):828–9.
3. Vestergaard ME, Macaskill P, Holt PE, et al. Dermoscopy compared with naked eye examination for the diagnosis of primary melanoma: a meta-analysis of studies performed in a clinical setting. Br J Dermatol 2008;159(3):669–76.
4. Menzies SW, Emery J, Staples M, et al. Impact of dermoscopy and short-term sequential digital dermoscopy imaging for the management of pigmented lesions in primary care: a sequential intervention trial. Br J Dermatol 2009;161(6):1270–7.
5. Carli P, De Giorgi V, Crocetti E, et al. Improvement of malignant/benign ratio in excised melanocytic lesions in the 'dermoscopy era': a retrospective study 1997-2001. Br J Dermatol 2004;150(4):687–92.
6. Tromme I, Sacré L, Hammouch F, et al. Availability of digital dermoscopy in daily practice dramatically reduces the number of excised melanocytic lesions: results from an observational study. Br J Dermatol 2012;167(4):778–86.
7. Sawyers EA, Wigle DT, Marghoob AA, et al. Dermoscopy training effect on diagnostic accuracy of skin lesions in Canadian family medicine physicians using the

triage amalgamated dermoscopic algorithm. Dermatol Pract Concept 2020; 10(2):e2020035.

8. Yélamos O, Braun RP, Liopyris K, et al. Dermoscopy and dermatopathology correlates of cutaneous neoplasms. J Am Acad Dermatol 2019;80(2):341–63.

9. Woltsche N, Schmid-Zalaudek K, Deinlein T, et al. Abundance of the benign melanocytic universe: Dermoscopic-histopathological correlation in nevi. J Dermatol 2017;44(5):499–506.

10. Errichetti E, Patriarca MM, Stinco G. Dermoscopy of congenital melanocytic nevi: a ten-year follow-up study and comparative analysis with acquired melanocytic nevi arising in prepubertal age. Eur J Dermatol 2017;27(5):505–10.

11. Argenziano G, Scalvenzi M, Staibano S, et al. Dermatoscopic pitfalls in differentiating pigmented Spitz naevi from cutaneous melanomas. Br J Dermatol 1999; 141(5):788–93.

12. Pizzichetta MA, Argenziano G, Grandi G, et al. Morphologic changes of a pigmented Spitz nevus assessed by dermoscopy. J Am Acad Dermatol 2002; 47(1):137–9.

13. Steiner A, Pehamberger H, Binder M, et al. Pigmented Spitz nevi: improvement of the diagnostic accuracy by epiluminescence microscopy. J Am Acad Dermatol 1992;27(5 Pt 1):697–701.

14. Vourc'h-Jourdain M, Martin L, Barbarot S, aRED. Large congenital melanocytic nevi: therapeutic management and melanoma risk: a systematic review. J Am Acad Dermatol 2013;68(3):493–8.

15. Seidenari S, Pellacani G, Martella A, et al. Instrument-, age- and site-dependent variations of dermoscopic patterns of congenital melanocytic naevi: a multicentre study. Br J Dermatol 2006;155(1):56–61.

16. Changchien L, Dusza SW, Agero AL, et al. Age- and site-specific variation in the dermoscopic patterns of congenital melanocytic nevi: an aid to accurate classification and assessment of melanocytic nevi. Arch Dermatol 2007;143(8): 1007–14.

17. Sakamoto S, Oiso N, Narita T, et al. Blue nevus with a dermoscopic appearance of peripheral streaks with branches. Case Rep Dermatol 2014;6(1):66–8.

18. Marghoob Ashfaq, Braun Ralph, editors. An atlas of dermoscopy. CRC Press; 2012.

19. Argenziano G, Catricalà C, Ardigo M, et al. Seven-point checklist of dermoscopy revisited. Br J Dermatol 2011;164(4):785–90.

20. Massi D, De Giorgi V, Soyer HP. Histopathologic correlates of dermoscopic criteria. Dermatol Clin 2001;19(2):259–68.

21. Gallegos-Hernández JF, Ortiz-Maldonado AL, Minauro-Muñoz GG, et al. Dermatoscopia en melanoma cutáneo [Dermoscopy in cutaneous melanoma]. Cir Cir 2015;83(2):107–11.

22. Menzies SW, Kreusch J, Byth K, et al. Dermoscopic evaluation of amelanotic and hypomelanotic melanoma. Arch Dermatol 2008;144(9):1120–7.

23. Soyer HP, Argenziano G, Chimenti S, et al. Dermoscopy of pigmented skin lesions. Eur J Dermatol 2001;11(3):270–7.

24. Scrivener Y, Grosshans E, Cribier B. Variations of basal cell carcinomas according to gender, age, location and histopathological subtype. Br J Dermatol 2002; 147(1):41–7.

25. Cameron MC, Lee E, Hibler BP, et al. Basal cell carcinoma: epidemiology; pathophysiology; clinical and histological subtypes; and disease associations. J Am Acad Dermatol 2019;80(2):303–17.

26. Marghoob A, Jaimes N. Basal cell carcinoma. Dermoscopedia. June 8, 2019, 11:10 UTC. Available at: https://dermoscopedia.org/w/index.php?title=Basal_cell_carcinoma&oldid=16531. Accessed September 16, 2020.

27. Yélamos O, Braun RP, Liopyris K, et al. Usefulness of dermoscopy to improve the clinical and histopathologic diagnosis of skin cancers. J Am Acad Dermatol 2019;80(2):365–77.

28. R. Strawberry pattern. Dermoscopedia. May 24, 2019, 15:34 UTC. Available at: https://dermoscopedia.org/w/index.php?title=Strawberry_pattern&oldid=16190. Accessed September 16, 2020.

29. R. Rosettes. Dermoscopedia. May 21, 2019, 09:29 UTC. Available at: https://dermoscopedia.org/w/index.php?title=Rosettes&oldid=15859. Accessed September 16, 2020.

30. Dimitriou F, Deinlein T, Zalaudek I. Bowen's disease. Dermoscopedia. June 8, 2019, 11:23 UTC. Available at: https://dermoscopedia.org/w/index.php?title=Bowen%27s_disease&oldid=16542. Accessed September 16, 2020.

31. Dimitriou F, Deinlein T, Zalaudek I. Squamous cell carcinoma. Dermoscopedia. June 8, 2019, 11:25 UTC. Available at: https://dermoscopedia.org/w/index.php?title=Squamous_cell_carcinoma&oldid=16543. Accessed September 17, 2020.

32. Lee WJ, Jung JM, Won CH, et al. Clinical and histological patterns of dermatofibroma without gross skin surface change: A comparative study with conventional dermatofibroma. Indian J Dermatol Venereol Leprol 2015;81(3):263–9.

33. Senel E. Dermatoscopy of non-melanocytic skin tumors. Indian J Dermatol Venereol Leprol 2011;77(1):16–22.

34. Karadag AS, Parish LC. The status of the seborrheic keratosis. Clin Dermatol 2018;36(2):275–7.

35. Papageorgiou C, Spyridis I, Manoli SM, et al. Accuracy of dermoscopic criteria for the differential diagnosis between irritated seborrheic keratosis and squamous cell carcinoma [published online ahead of print, 2020 Feb 14]. J Am Acad Dermatol 2020;S0190-9622(20):30227–9.

36. Wollina U. Recent advances in managing and understanding seborrheic keratosis. F1000Res 2019;8:F1000. Faculty Rev-1520.

37. Gülseren D, Hofmann-Wellenhof R. Evaluation of dermoscopic criteria for seborrheic keratosis on non-polarized versus polarized dermoscopy. Skin Res Technol 2019;25(6):801–4.

38. Lin J, Han S, Cui L, et al. Evaluation of dermoscopic algorithm for seborrhoeic keratosis: a prospective study in 412 patients. J Eur Acad Dermatol Venereol 2014;28(7):957–62.

39. Braun RP, Ludwig S, Marghoob AA. Differential diagnosis of seborrheic keratosis: clinical and dermoscopic features. J Drugs Dermatol 2017;16(9):835–42.

40. Qadeer HA, Singal A, Patel BC. Cherry hemangioma. 2020. In: StatPearls [Internet]. Treasure Island (FL: StatPearls Publishing; 2020.

41. Rogers T, Marino M, Dusza SW, et al. Triage amalgamated dermoscopic algorithm (TADA) for skin cancer screening. Dermatol Pract Concept 2017;7(2): 39–46.

42. Seiverling EV, Ahrns HT, Greene A, et al. Teaching Benign Skin Lesions as a Strategy to Improve the Triage Amalgamated Dermoscopic Algorithm (TADA). J Am Board Fam Med 2019;32(1):96–102.

43. Marghboob AA, Malvehy J, Braun RP. Atlas of dermoscopy. 2nd ed. Boca Raton: CRC Press;; 2011.

Large and Intermediate Joint Injections

Olecranon Bursa, Greater Trochanteric Bursa, Medial and Lateral Epicondyle Peritendinous Injections

Kimberly Kaiser, MD[a],*, Michael Fitzgerald, DO[b,1],
Brady Fleshman, MD[c], Kathleen Roberts, MD[d]

KEYWORDS

- Greater trochanter bursitis • Olecranon bursitis • Medial epicondylosis
- Lateral epicondylosis

KEY POINTS

- Olecranon bursitis is an inflammatory condition caused by repetitive microtrauma to the posterior elbow and is usually treated conservatively. When septic bursitis is suspected, bursal aspiration can be performed.
- Greater trochanteric bursitis patients present with lateral hip pain and commonly improve with physical therapy, activity modification, weight loss, and occasionally corticosteroid injections.
- Medial and lateral epicondylosis are degenerative processes of the flexor and extensor muscles of the forearm, respectively, and are usually amenable to activity modification, physical therapy, and occasionally corticosteroid injections.

OLECRANON BURSA INJECTION

Introduction/History/Definitions/Background

- Olecranon bursitis is an inflammatory condition characterized by abnormal fluid accumulation within the olecranon bursal cavity, a synovial membrane located immediately posterior to the olecranon bone of the elbow.[1]

No authors have any commercial or financial conflicts of interest.
[a] Department of Orthopaedic Surgery and Sports Medicine, University of Kentucky, 740S Limestone, K400, Lexington, KY 40536, USA; [b] Department of Family and Community Medicine, University of Kentucky, 4200 N. Division Ave., Comstock Park, MI 49321, USA; [c] Department of Orthopedic Surgery and Sports Medicine, University of Missouri, 7115 E St Charles Road, Columbia, MO 65202, USA; [d] Department of Family and Community Medicine, University of Kentucky, 2195 Harrodsburg Road, Suite 125, Lexington, KY 40504, USA
[1] Present address: 2630 Middleboro Lane Northeast, Grand Rapids, MI 49506
* Corresponding author.
E-mail address: kim.kaiser@uky.edu

Nature of the Problem/Diagnosis

- Commonly caused by repetitive microtrauma to the posterior elbow.[2]
- Described as aseptic (noninfective) or septic (infective, most commonly by *Staphylococcus aureus*).[1]
- Aseptic causes are categorized as acute (direct trauma) or chronic (systemic and rheumatologic disorders including gout, rheumatoid arthritis, and long-term hemodialysis).
  - Of all bursae, the olecranon bursa is the most affected by inflammatory processes.[3]

Anatomy

- Superficial, closed synovial sac that allows the bony olecranon to glide smoothly across overlying tissues with flexion and extension of the elbow.
- Localized deep to the skin of the elbow, superficial to the insertion of the triceps tendon at the olecranon process of the ulna.
- Especially susceptible to trauma and infection due to its superficial location and limited vascularity.[1]

Clinical Presentation

- Aseptic bursitis often presents as painless swelling over the posterior elbow. Aseptic bursitis is frequently found in manual laborers who spend prolonged periods of time with direct pressure on their elbows (ie, plumbers, miners, electricians)[2] (**Fig. 1**).
- In septic cases, the posterior elbow may be erythematous, warm, and tender to the touch with or without systemic symptoms of infection (fever, malaise, nausea, and so forth).

Observation/Assessment/Evaluation

- Diagnosis is largely clinical and is based on history and examination.
- Differential diagnosis includes septic and inflammatory arthritis, cellulitis, and Morel-Lavallee lesions.[2]
- Consider plain radiograph films with recent trauma or suspected foreign body.
- Ultrasonography helps determine bursal involvement with significant soft tissue swelling.
- If septic cause is suspected, aspiration and analysis of the bursal fluid is the gold standard.[2]

Preoperative/Preprocedure Planning

- Indications for aspiration: diagnostic evaluation, symptomatic relief, therapeutic intervention
- Contraindications for aspiration: aspiration through overlying cellulitis or in the setting of acute olecranon fracture[4]

Prep and Patient Positioning

- Inform the patient of procedural specifics including purpose, risks, benefits, and alternatives.
- Obtain informed consent.
- Supplies:
  - 18-gauge, 1.5-inch needle
  - 10 cc syringe

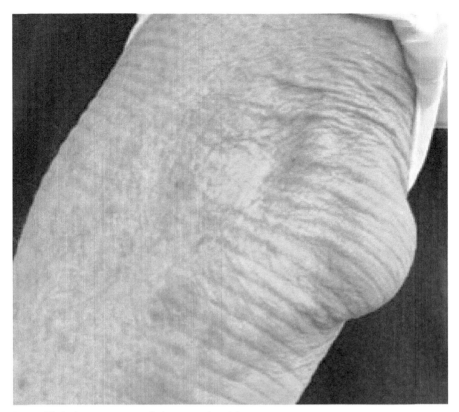

Fig. 1. Clinical appearance of olecranon bursitis.

- Position the patient seated with their elbow at 90°, arm raised above the shoulder, and forearm resting on a sterile surface.
- Cleanse the skin of the posterior elbow with an antiseptic solution (eg, chlorhexidine, betadine).
- Ethyl chloride spray may be used for topical anesthesia.
  - Note: lidocaine is generally avoided due to the superficial location of the bursa and risk for skewing the fluid analysis results.[4]

Procedural Approach

- Provide distal traction to the adjacent skin of the forearm to create a Z-shaped needle track when traction is released.[2]
- Using an 18-gauge 1.5-inch needle and 10 cc syringe, puncture the skin of the posterior elbow directing the needle distally (parallel to the ulna).
- Apply gentle traction to the plunger to aspirate the bursal contents.
- On completion, remove the needle and release skin traction on the forearm.
- Discard the needle and apply a sterile bandage and compression dressing.
- Send the bursal fluid for cell count with differential, Gram stain, culture, and crystal analysis.[4]

Recovery and Rehabilitation

- Advise the patient to keep the area clean, dry, and covered and avoid submersing the elbow for 48 to 72 hours to reduce the risk for postprocedure infection.

- Complications are rare but include bleeding, local nerve damage, and introducing superficial infection into a previously sterile bursa.[4]

Management

- Acute, aseptic bursitis is managed conservatively with rest, ice, compression, nonsteroidal anti-inflammatory drugs (NSAIDs), activity modification, and posterior elbow padding.[2]
- Corticosteroid injection is not recommended due to high risk of iatrogenic infection (10%) and recurrence rate (25% at 8 weeks).[5]
- A 2014 systematic review found that conservative management is safer and more effective due to higher rate of clinical resolution and lower rates of overall complications, persistent drainage, and bursal infection than bursectomy for chronic olecranon bursitis.[6]
- Moreover, corticosteroid injection for aseptic bursitis is associated with significant risk without improving clinical outcomes.[6]
- Empirical management of uncomplicated septic olecranon bursitis results in full recovery and low recurrence without the need for surgical bursectomy.[7]

Outcome

- Aseptic olecranon bursitis is generally benign and self-limited.
  - Anatomic and structural variants, such as olecranon bone spurs, may increase the risk of recurrence.[3]
- Septic bursitis only rarely progresses to systemic disease.

Summary

- Olecranon bursitis is a common cause of posterior elbow swelling.
- Aseptic cases are typically benign and self-limited, whereas septic cases require more careful evaluation and management.
- Although bursal aspiration and fluid analysis remains the gold standard for diagnosis of septic bursitis, new evidence suggests empirical antibiotic therapy may be an effective and safe treatment alternative.
- Corticosteroid injection for chronic aseptic bursitis is not indicated due to poor efficacy and risk of infection.

Clinics Care Points

- Bursal aspiration with fluid analysis should be performed in patients with suspected septic superficial bursitis. (SORT C)[2]
- Initial management of superficial bursitis caused by microtrauma should consist of conservative measures such as padding, ice, elevation, and analgesics (only for pain) (SORT B).[2]
- Septic superficial bursitis should be treated empirically with systemic antibiotics covering *S aureus* and *Streptococcus pyogenes*. The antibiotic regimen can be modified, if needed, after culture and sensitivity results from aspirated bursal fluids are available (SORT B).[2]

GREATER TROCHANTERIC BURSA INJECTION
Introduction/History/Definitions/Background

- Greater trochanteric pain syndrome (GTPS), also referred to as greater trochanteric bursitis, is typically a self-limiting disorder involving pain in the lateral hip.

Nature of the Problem/Diagnosis

- Historically, the pathophysiology of GTPS was thought to be secondary to inflammation from the trochanteric bursa. However, trochanteric bursitis is somewhat of a misnomer because inflammation is not commonly found. GTPS includes several causes including gluteal tendinopathy, gluteal tears, bursitis, iliotibial band (ITB) and tensor fascia lata (TFL) tension, and external coxa saltans (ie, external snapping hip).[8,9]

Anatomy

- Muscles that attach to the greater trochanter include the gluteus medius and minimus, piriformis, obturator externus and internus, superior and inferior gemellus, and quadratus femoris.
  ○ The gluteus medius and gluteus minimus are the primary lateral attachments to the greater trochanter.
- The gluteus maximus is the most superficial gluteal muscle and has a broad distal attachment to the TFL and femur. It does not insert directly on the greater trochanter.
- There are typically 3 bursae lateral to the greater trochanter. The largest is termed the subgluteus maximus bursa, also commonly referred to as the "trochanteric bursa."
- The gluteus medius attaches to the lateral and superoposterior facet. The gluteus minimus attaches to the anterior facet.

Clinical Presentation

- Often described as lateral hip pain exacerbated by active abduction and passive adduction.[8]
- Pain with direct palpation or lying on affected side while sleeping.
- Lateral hip pain with prolonged sitting.

Observation/Assessment/Evaluation

- Pain with direct palpation over greater trochanter
- Trendelenburg gait
- Hip abductor weakness
- Positive FABER

Preoperative/Preprocedure Planning

- This planning is best done when patient is ambulatory enough to lie on an examination table (ie, not wheelchair bound).

Prep and Patient Positioning

- Inform the patient of procedural specifics including purpose, risks, benefits, and alternatives.
- Obtain informed consent.
- Supplies:
  ○ 21- to 25-gauge, 1.5-inch needle for thin patients or 3.5-inch spinal needle used for larger, obese patients
  ○ 10 cc syringe
  ○ Injectate: combination of 4 cc 1% lidocaine without epinephrine, 4 cc 0.5% bupivacaine, and 2 cc 40 mg/mL Kenalog

- Note: other formulations are efficacious (eg, 2 cc lidocaine, 2 cc bupivacaine, and 1 cc 40 mg/mL Kenalog) and up to provider preference based on patient comorbidities
- Position: lateral decubitus with affected side up.
- Ethyl chloride spray may be used for topical anesthesia.

Procedural Approach

- Identify 2 bony landmarks. The superior landmark is the iliac crest and inferior to this is the greater trochanter (**Fig. 2**).
- Use your fingers to identify where the greater trochanter bone is closest to the skin and mark this location. This should also be on or in close proximity to the patient's area of greatest tenderness.
- Cleanse the skin with antiseptic solution (eg, chlorhexidine, betadine).
- Orient needle perpendicular to the ground.
- Insert needle through the skin until you feel contact with lateral aspect of femur bone.
- Draw needle back slightly (approximately 2–4 mm) in normal sized adult.
- Inject solution. If experiencing resistance, medication is likely within gluteus tendon. Either slightly advance or draw back the needle 1 to 2 mm until solution is more easily injected.
- Discard needle and apply a sterile bandage.

Recovery and Rehabilitation (Including Postprocedure Care)

- A driver is not typically required following the procedure.
- Avoid submerging the injection site for the next 48 to 72 hours.
- Injections into the trochanteric bursa are relatively safe. There is a small risk of skin irritation, swelling, and a temporary increase in local pain.[8]

Management

- Nonoperative management with activity modification, NSAIDs, physical therapy, weight loss, and/or corticosteroid injections (CSIs) can be expected to successfully treat greater than 90% of all cases.[8]

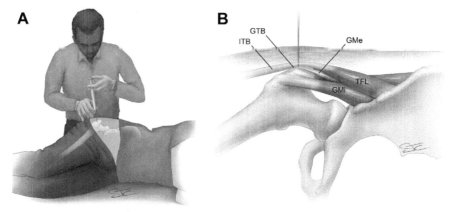

Fig. 2. (*A*) Greater trochanter injection patient and physician positioning. (*B*) Focused anatomic view of greater trochanter injection. ITB, iliotibial band; GTB, greater trochanter bursa (ie, subgluteus maximus bursa); GMe, gluteus medius; GMi, gluteus minimus; TFL, tensor fasciae latae. (© Copyright 2021 by The Curators of the University of Missouri, a public corporation.)

- Home exercise programs should focus on gluteal, hip abductor, and quadriceps strengthening.
- Recurrence is common.
- Surgical management options include repair of gluteal tears, longitudinal ITB release, ITB Z-plasty, bursectomy, and osteotomy.[8,10]
  - Technique: open or endoscopic

Outcomes

- Resolution of symptoms and return to activity after a CSI ranges from 49% to 100%.[8]
  - 33% of patients received a second injection and some as many as 5.[8]
- CSI had superior outcomes for improvements in pain and functional and quality-of-life measures compared with other conservative modalities for up to 3 months.[11]

Summary

- GTPS is a likely culprit when patients present with lateral hip pain worse with palpation or lying on the affected side and no radiographic evidence of osteoarthritis.
- CSI into the greater trochanteric bursa is a safe procedure that can be completed in the office with relatively few adverse effects during or after the procedure.
- Repeat injections are sometimes needed. Consider a multimodal approach to GTPS, particularly if symptoms are recurring or a second injection is required.

Clinics Care Points

- GTPS can be distinguished from hip osteoarthritis by an ability to walk for a duration greater than 30 minutes, ease of manipulation of shoes and socks, and lateral hip pain with FABER test.[12]
- Home training, single steroid injection, and radial shock wave treatment have differing success rates. Outcomes measured included degree of recovery measured on a 6-point Likert scale with treatment success defined as subjects rating completely recovered or much improved. The home training included piriformis and ITB stretching and quadriceps and gluteal strengthening. They performed these exercises twice daily for 12 weeks. At 1, 4, and 15 months, CSI had a success rate of 75%, 51%, and 48%, respectively; home training had a success rate of 7%, 41%, and 80%, respectively; and radial shock wave therapy had a success rate of 13%, 68%, and 74%, respectively.[13]

MEDIAL AND LATERAL EPICONDYLE PERITENDINOUS INJECTIONS
Introduction/History/Definitions/Background

- Medial and lateral epicondylosis (golfer's elbow and tennis elbow, respectively) are disorders of the elbow that include both functional impairment as well as chronic pain with the medial exacerbated by wrist flexion and the lateral by wrist extension activities.

Nature of the Problem/Diagnosis

- The pathophysiology of epicondylosis is a degenerative process of the flexor and extensor muscles of the forearm with the development of microscopic tears, resulting in calcification, fibrosis, and a less functional tendon. Medial epicondylosis originates from frequent stress of the muscles used for wrist flexion and forearm pronation, whereas lateral epicondylosis originates from frequent stress of the extensor carpi radialis brevis.[14]

Anatomy

- The lateral humeral epicondyle is the attachment point of the common extensor origin consisting of 5 muscles:
  - Extensor carpi radialis longus
  - Extensor carpi radialis brevis
  - Extensor digitorum communis
  - Extensor digiti minimi
  - Extensor carpi ulnaris
- The medial humeral epicondyle is the attachment point for the flexor-pronator muscle group:
  - Pronator teres
  - Flexor carpi radialis
- There are also multiple adjacent structures to the medial epicondyle including the ulnar nerve, the medial antebrachial cutaneous nerve, and the ulnar collateral ligament.

Clinical Presentation

- Lateral epicondylosis:
  - Lateral elbow pain
  - Pain with wrist extension
  - Weakened grip strength
- Medial epicondylosis:
  - Medial elbow pain
  - Pain with wrist flexion and pronation
  - Weakened grip strength

Observation/Assessment/Evaluation

- Pain with direct palpation over the medial or lateral epicondyle
- Medial epicondylosis:
  - Pain with resisted wrist pronation
  - Pain with resisted wrist flexion
- Lateral epicondylosis:
  - Pain with resisted wrist supination
  - Pain with resisted wrist extension
  - Pain with resisted third finger extension

Preoperative/Preprocedure Planning

- For the lateral epicondyle peritendinous injection: this should be done in a location where the patient is able to be seated in a chair with side rails and the elbow is rested on the examination table.
- For the medial epicondyle peritendinous injection: this should be done in a location where the patient is able to lay supine in a comfortable position.
- Counsel the patient that their pain may worsen over the subsequent 24 to 48 hours; however, it should resolve after that time.

Prep and Patient Positioning

- Inform the patient of procedural specifics including purpose, risks, benefits, and alternatives.
- Obtain informed consent.
- Supplies:
  - 25-gauge, 1-inch needle

- ○ 5 cc syringe
- ○ Injectate: combination of 1 cc 1% lidocaine without epinephrine and 1 cc 80 mg/mL Depo-Medrol.
  - • Note: other formulations are efficacious and up to provider preference based on patient's comorbidities.
- • Position for lateral epicondyle peritendinous injection: seated in a chair with side rails and back, shoulder flexed to 90°, and elbow flexed at 90° and resting on the examination table.
- • Position for medial epicondyle peritendinous injection: supine on the examination table with arm in an abducted position, ideally with the hand under the head with the elbow flexed to 90°.
- • Ethyl chloride spray may be used for topical anesthesia (see **Fig. 2**).

Procedural Approach

Lateral epicondyle peritendinous injection

- • Identify the lateral epicondyle of the elbow and the point of maximal tenderness at the insertion of the common extensor tendon. Mark this location (**Fig. 3**).
- • Cleanse the skin with antiseptic solution (eg, chlorhexidine, betadine).
- • Orient needle perpendicular to the lateral epicondyle.
- • Insert the needle into the skin until you hit the bone of the lateral epicondyle and then withdraw the needle slightly.
- • Gently fan the contents of the syringe into the subcutaneous tissue.
- • There should be very little resistance to the injection. If encountering resistance, draw back 1 to 2 mm to avoid injecting the medication directly into the tendon.

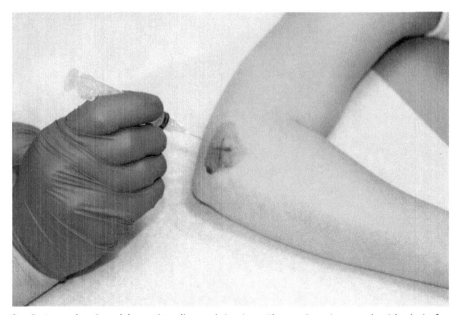

Fig. 3. Lateral epicondyle peritendinous injection. The patient is seated with their feet resting on the floor and their elbow flexed at 90°. The point of maximal tenderness at the lateral epicondyle has been marked and prepped with antiseptic solution. A 25-gauge 1-inch needle is being inserted at a perpendicular angle with 1 mL of 80 mg/mL Depo-Medrol and 1 mL of 1% lidocaine.

- Discard the needle and apply a sterile bandage.[15]

Medial epicondyle peritendinous injection

- Identify the medial epicondyle of the elbow and the point of maximal tenderness at the insertion of the common flexor tendon. Mark this location (**Fig. 4**).
- Of note the ulnar nerve should not be able to be palpated from this position, as it should be deep to the epicondyle.
- Cleanse the skin with antiseptic solution (eg, chlorhexidine, betadine).
- Orient needle perpendicular to the medial epicondyle.
- Insert the needle into the skin until you make contact with the bone of the medial epicondyle and then withdraw the needle slightly.
- Gently fan the contents of the syringe into the subcutaneous tissue.
- There should be very little resistance to the injection. If encountering resistance, draw back 1 to 2 mm to avoid injecting the medication directly into the tendon.
- Discard the needle and apply a sterile bandage.[16]

Recovery and Rehabilitation

- Patients should be counseled to not lift greater than 5 to 10 pounds on the affected side for 3 to 5 days following the injection to help reduce the risk of tendon rupture.
- Avoid submerging the site of injection for the next 48 to 72 hours.
- Injections into the medial and lateral epicondyle peritendinous area are relatively safe. There is a small risk of infection (which is reduced by using aseptic

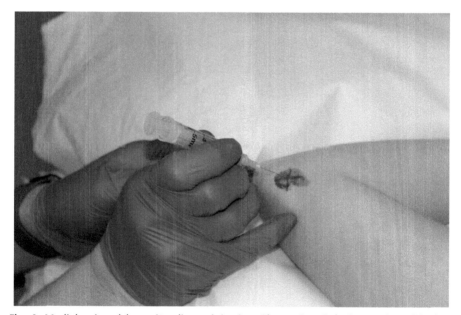

Fig. 4. Medial epicondyle peritendinous injection. The patient is laying supine with their elbow flexed at 90°. The point of maximal tenderness at the medial epicondyle has been marked and prepped with antiseptic solution. The ulnar nerve has been located and isolated. A 25-gauge 1-inch needle is being inserted at a perpendicular angle with 1 mL of 80 mg/mL Depo-Medrol and 1 mL of 1% lidocaine.

technique), tendon rupture, ulnar nerve injury with medial epicondyle injections, and a temporary increase in local pain in around 25% of patients.[15,16]

Management

- Initial treatment should begin with nonoperative management that includes activity modification, physical therapy, medications such as NSAIDs, and corticosteroid injections. This has been shown to treat lateral epicondylosis (defined as the resolution of symptoms) in 95% of cases and medial epicondylosis in 85% to 95% of patients.[17]
- Surgical management for lateral epicondylosis involves release of the pathologic tendon from its origin at the lateral epicondyle with debridement of the affected tissue. The bony surface can also be scored to help stimulate healing as well.[17]
  - Technique: open, percutaneous, arthroscopic
- Surgical management for medial epicondylosis involves debridement of the common flexor pronator tendon with the pathologic portion excised and the healthy portion reattached.[17]
  - Technique: open, percutaneous, arthroscopic

Outcomes

- Treatment of lateral epicondylosis with corticosteroid injection is effective for pain relief and improvement in function in the short term (less than 12 weeks).[18]
- Reported recurrence rates are up to 37% at 6 months following corticosteroid injection.[18]
- Treatment of medial epicondylosis with corticosteroid injection is effective in acute improvement in pain relief at 6 weeks compared with no injection; however, by 3 months reported pain was similar between the 2 groups.[19]

Summary

- Medial and lateral epicondylosis are 2 of the most common causes of elbow pain and functional deficits of the wrist and forearm in the general, working, and athletic populations.
- Corticosteroid injections as a conservative treatment option for medial and lateral epicondylosis is an option for acute pain relief in both conditions that are associated with very few adverse effects.
- To achieve long-term pain relief, corticosteroid injections should be combined with a formal physical therapy plan including home exercises with surgery only needed in around 5% to 8% of total cases.[17,20]

Clinics Care Points

- Although lateral epicondylosis is commonly referred to as "tennis elbow," tennis players make up only 10% of this patient population.[20]
- Medial epicondylosis is a clinical diagnosis and is more difficult to discern. Ulnar neuritis and ulnar collateral ligament injury commonly masquerade as or occur concomitantly with this condition.[17]

ACKNOWLEDGMENTS

Special thanks to Stacy Turpin Cheavens, MS, Certified Medical Illustrator, for her contributions to this article.

REFERENCES

1. Blackwell J, Hay BA, Bolt AM, et al. Olecranon Bursitis: a Systematic Overview. Shoulder Elbow 2014;6:182–90.
2. Khodaee M. Common Superficial Bursitis. Am Fam Physician 2017;95:224–31.
3. Reilly D, Kamineni S. Olecranon Bursitis. J Shoulder Elbow Surg 2016;25:158–67.
4. O'Shea N, Tadi P. Olecranon Bursa Aspiration. In: StatPearls. Treasure Island (FL): StatPearls Publishing; 2021. Accessed April 22, 2021.
5. Pangia J, Rizvi T. Olecranon bursitis. In: StatPearls. Treasure Island (FL): StatPearls Publishing; 2020. Accessed April 22, 2021.
6. Sayegh E, Strauch R. Treatment of Olecranon Bursitis: a Systematic Review. Arch Orthop Trauma Surg 2014;134:1517–36.
7. Deal JB, Vaslow AS, Bickley RJ, et al. Empirical Treatment of Uncomplicated Septic Olecranon Bursitis Without Aspiration. J Hand Surg 2020;45:20–5.
8. Lustenberger D, Ng V, Best T. Efficacy of treatment of Trochanteric Bursitis: A systematic review. Clin J Sport Med 2011;21:447–53.
9. Mallow M, Nazarian L. Greater trochanteric pain syndrome diagnosis and treatment. Phys Med Rehabil Clin N Am 2014;25:279–89.
10. Redmond J, Chen A, Domb B. Greater Trochanteric Pain Syndrome. J Am Acad Orthop Surg 2016;24:231–40.
11. Barratt P, Brookes N, Newson A. Conservative treatments for greater trochanteric pain syndrome: A systematic review. Physiotherapy 2017;103. https://doi.org/10.1016/j.physio.2017.11.010.
12. Fearon A, Scarvell J, Neeman T, et al. Greater trochanteric pain syndrome: Defining the clinical syndrome. Br J Sports Med 2012;47:649–53.
13. Rompe J, Segal N, Cacchio A, et al. Home training, local corticosteroid injection, or radial shock wave therapy for greater trochanter pain syndrome. Am J Sports Med 2009;37:1981–90.
14. Tarpada S, Morris T, Lian J, et al. Current Advances in the Treatment of Medial and Lateral Epicondylitis. J Orthop 2018;15:107–10.
15. Waldman S. Lateral Epicondyle Injection. In: Atlas of pain management injection techniques. 2017. pp. 189-193).
16. Waldman S. Medial Epicondyle Injection for Golfer's Elbow. In: Atlas of pain management injection techniques. 2017. pp. 189-193.
17. Fleck K, Field E, Field L. Lateral and Medial Epicondylitis in the Athlete. Oper Tech Sports Med 2017;25:269–78.
18. Houck D, Kraeutler M, Thornton L, et al. Treatment of Lateral Epicondylitis with Autologous Blood, Platelet-Rich Plasma, or Corticosteroid Injections: A Systematic Review of Overlapping Meta-analyses. Orthop J Sports Med 2019;7(3). 2325967119831052.
19. Stahl S, Kaufman T. The Efficacy of an Injection of Steroids for Medial Epicondylitis. J Bone Joint Surg Am 1997;79:1648–52.
20. De Smedt T, De Jong A, Van Leemput W, et al. Lateral epicondylitis in tennis: Update on aetiology, biomechanics and treatment. Br J Sports Med 2007;41:816–9.

Small Joint, Tendon, and Myofascial Injections

Lindsay Lafferty, MD[a,b], Smriti Gupta, MD[c], Ashley Koontz, DO[a], Cayce Onks, DO, MS, ATC[a,b],*

KEYWORDS

- Injection • Carpal tunnel • de Quervain • Trigger finger • Ganglion • Trigger point
- Plantar fascia

KEY POINTS

- Small joint, peritendinous, and myofascial injections can be used for both diagnostic and therapeutic purposes.
- Understanding of anatomy before injection and identification of pertinent local landmarks is critical.
- Patient consent should include potential benefits, complications, and side effects.
- Injectable anesthetics are typically effective within seconds to minutes, and duration of effect varies depending on the anesthetic used.
- Injectable steroids vary in time to onset. Most of the patients note symptom relief within weeks, with average effects lasting 3 months.

INTRODUCTION

Injections and aspirations are used for both diagnostic and therapeutic purposes.[1] Preprocedure planning is essential to provide a safe and effective treatment, and this includes understanding absolute and relative contraindications for the procedure. These contraindications may vary based on the structure being injected and the comorbidities of your patient. Equipment may vary depending on the injection being performed and should be gathered before beginning the procedure. Informed consent should be obtained including potential complications and side effects. It is critical to have a complete understanding of the pertinent anatomy before injection and be able to identify pertinent local landmarks.[2] Care should be taken to minimize risk of infection before injection. Evidence is limited for guidance on medication dose and postprocedure protocols. Here the authors review general guidance for soft tissue

[a] Department of Family and Community Medicine, Penn State Health, 500 University Drive, Hershey, PA 17033, USA; [b] Department of Orthopedics and Rehabilitation, Penn State Health, 500 University Drive, Hershey, PA 17033, USA; [c] Department of Family and Community Medicine, Penn State Health, 1850 East Park Avenue Suite 207, State College, PA 16803, USA
* Corresponding author. Department of Family and Community Medicine, Penn State Health, 500 University Drive, Hershey, PA 17033, USA
E-mail address: conks@pennstatehealth.psu.edu

Prim Care Clin Office Pract 49 (2022) 131–143
https://doi.org/10.1016/j.pop.2021.10.006
0095-4543/22/© 2021 Elsevier Inc. All rights reserved.

and joint injections followed by specific guidance for carpal tunnel, first dorsal compartment, trigger finger, ganglion cysts, trigger point, and plantar fascia.

GENERAL SOFT TISSUE AND JOINT INJECTION INDICATIONS

Injections and aspirations are used for both diagnostic and therapeutic purposes.[1]

Diagnostic

- Introduction of local anesthetic into a joint to provide pain relief, allowing a more comprehensive examination.[3]
- Therapeutic trial to differentiate various causes of pain.[1]
- Aspiration to evaluate synovial fluid for infection, trauma, and rheumatoid and crystal arthropathy.[3,4]

Therapeutic

- Aspiration to remove tense effusions, relieve pain, and improve function.[1,3,5]
- Introduction of intraarticular steroid for treatment of inflammation, crystalloid arthropathies, inflammatory arthritis, and osteoarthrosis.[1,5]
- Soft tissue indications for injection include bursitis, tendinosis, trigger points, ganglion cysts, neuromas, nerve entrapment syndromes, and fasciitis.[5]

CONTRAINDICATIONS

Absolute contraindications to injections include the following[1–3,5]:
- History of allergy or anaphylaxis to injected solutions
- Injection through overlying skin breakdown or infection
- Injection around prosthetic joint due to risk of infection
- Corticosteroid injection in a joint with intraarticular fracture
- Corticosteroid injection into tendons due to risk of tendon rupture

Relative contraindications include the following[1–3,5]:
- Uncontrolled diabetes, as corticosteroids may result in temporary elevation in blood glucose
- Immunosuppression
- History of avascular necrosis
- Anticoagulation or uncontrolled coagulopathies
- Lack of response to prior similar injections

EQUIPMENT AND MATERIALS

- Cleansing solution (betadine, chlorhexidine, alcohol) (**Fig. 1**)
- Gloves
- Skin marker
- Sterile gauze
- Syringes
  - 1 to 10 cc syringes for injections
  - 3 to 60 cc syringes for aspirations
- Needles
  - 21- to 27-gauge 1.5 inch needles for injection
  - 18- to 20-gauge needles for aspirations and drawing mediation[1]
- Dressing
- Optional
  - Hemostat surgical clamp for switching syringes after aspiration and before injection

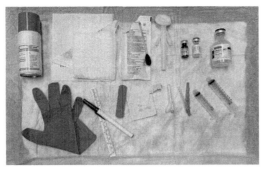

Fig. 1. Equipment and materials.

- ○ Topical analgesia
  - ■ Ethyl chloride topical spray, which rapidly cools skin
  - ■ EMLA cream, which must be applied at least 1 hour before injection[2]
- • Common Agents
  - ○ Local anesthetic
    - ■ Uses include diminishing pain, aiding in diagnosis, and providing volume for corticosteroid injections[1]
    - ■ Lidocaine (Xylocaine) 1% without epinephrine—short acting (3 hours)[1]
    - ■ Bupivacaine (Marcaine) 0.5%—long acting (6 hours)
  - ○ Corticosteroids
    - ■ Used to treat local inflammatory response
    - ■ Less soluble—favored for joint injections[4]
      - • Methylprednisolone acetate (Depo-Medrol)
      - • Triamcinolone acetonide (Kenalog)
      - • Triamcinolone hexacetonide (Aristospan)
    - ■ More soluble—favored for soft tissue injections[4]
      - • Betamethasone sodium phosphate (Celestone)
      - • Dexamethasone sodium phosphate (Decadron)
      - • Prednisolone sodium phosphate (Hydeltrasol)
    - ■ Dosage
      - • There isimited evidence-based guidance, but typically a small dose for small joints/soft tissue structures and can increase for moderate or large structures (triamcinolone range: 20mg–80 mg total dose range).

PREPROCEDURE PLANNING

Gather all equipment and materials needed for the procedure before beginning. Informed consent should be obtained before the procedure. The patient should be positioned comfortably, sitting or lying, and the provider should be able to assume a comfortable position to easily identify landmarks and administer the injection.[1]

It is critical to have a complete understanding of the anatomy in each area before injection and be able to identify pertinent local landmarks.[2] The injection technique should minimize risk of infection. The injection site should be marked and then prepped with appropriate antiseptic solution. Sterile needles and syringes should be used and when possible single dose vials of injectable medication. Needles should be changed after drawing up the solution before injection.[2] Always use universal precautions to avoid inadvertent contact with sharp objects, blood, or body fluids. When performing injections, the "no-touch" technique should be followed, meaning nothing is to contact the injection site after sterile preparation of the skin is completed.[3]

RECOVERY, REHABILITATION, AND OUTCOMES

- Use after injection
  - There is no evidence to guide postinjection protocols. Recommendations typically suggest refraining from strenuous activities that use the site of the injection for 24 to 48 hours. In particular, if injectable anesthetics have been used patients should wait until this effect has dissipated before engaging in activities that stress the injected area.
  - For peritendinous injections using steroids you may consider a longer period of relative rest due to concern of tendon weakening from the injection.
  - Infection precautions could include not submersing the injection site in water for 24 hours.
- Time to onset of injected medication:
  - Injectable anesthetics will be effective typically within seconds to minutes and their half-lives will vary with short-acting (3–4 hours) and long-acting (6–8 hours) options.
  - Injectable steroids vary in their time to onset, but most of the patients have symptom relief within weeks and on average the effects will last 3 months.

COMPLICATIONS AND SIDE EFFECTS

- Patient consent should include a conversation about potential complications and side effects.
  - Most common
    - Steroid flare (acute pain postinjection lasting hours to days)
    - Skin hypopigmentation
    - Fat necrosis
    - Hyperglycemia (more concerning in uncontrolled diabetics)
  - Rare
    - Infection
    - Tendon rupture
    - Chondrotoxicity
    - Osteonecrosis

CARPAL TUNNEL

Diagnosis: carpal tunnel syndrome is caused by entrapment of the median nerve as it passes under the flexor retinaculum of the ventral wrist.[6,7] It is most classically diagnosed clinically by consistent history and neuromuscular examination findings, such as a positive Phalen or Tinel testing.[6,7] The most common initial symptoms include paresthesia and pain of the hand at night or with repetitive use. Risk factors for carpal tunnel syndrome include diabetes, menopause, hypothyroidism, obesity, arthritis, and pregnancy.[6,7] Injection may be indicated if the patient has persistent pain that does not respond to standard conservative therapy, including splinting, activity modification, and physical therapy.

Anatomy: the carpal tunnel is a canal of the ventral wrist made from bones and ligaments to hold the flexor tendons and associated median nerve in place.[8] The medial border of the carpal tunnel is the hook of the hamate and pisiform. The lateral border is the trapezium and scaphoid. The rest of the carpal bones make up the dorsal border of the carpal tunnel, and the flexor retinaculum creates the ventral border of the carpal tunnel. Contained within the carpal tunnel are the flexor tendons of the fingers and thumb as well as the median nerve. The median nerve lies deep to and between the palmaris longus and flexor carpi ulnaris tendons at the level of the distal wrist crease. Asking the patient to bring their fifth finger to their thumb can help elevate these tendons for identification[8] (**Fig. 2**).

Preparation and Positioning

1. Gather the recommended supplies: cleansing solution, 25 to 27 gauge 1 to 1.5 inch needle, 5 mL syringe, injectate, gauze, adhesive bandage, and sterile skin marker.
2. Patient may be seated in front of a table or lying supine on an examination table. Place palm facing upward on table.
3. A small towel roll can be used as needed to place the wrist in a neutral position.
4. Prepare syringe with a 1:1 preparation of 0.5 to 1 mL of anesthetic and 0.5 to 1 mL of steroid solution with a 25- to 27-gauge needle. Dexamethasone is preferred for this superficial injection site to minimize risk for skin atrophy and discoloration.

Procedure

1. Identify the flexor carpi ulnaris, palmaris longus, and distal wrist crease along the flexor surface of the wrist (see **Fig. 2**). If the palmaris longus is absent, use the midline of the wrist.
2. Identify the space just ulnar to the palmaris longus at the proximal wrist crease. Use the skin marker to mark this location, which will be the injection site.
3. The injection site should be cleaned with appropriate antiseptic solution.
4. Insert the needle bevel up into marked site at a 30- to 45-degree angle just ulnar to the palmaris longus, angled toward the index finger and advance 1 to 2 cm.
5. If paresthesia is reported in the palm or fingers the needle should be withdrawn slightly and redirected in an ulnar direction.
6. Slowly inject solution into carpal tunnel space. If resistance is felt, slightly withdraw and redirect the needle to avoid intratendinous injection.
7. Remove needle, clean site, and provide postprocedure care.

FIRST DORSAL COMPARTMENT

Diagnosis: de Quervain tenosynovitis is a common cause of pain to the radial aspect of the wrist due to pathology within the first dorsal compartment of the hand. Repetitive microtrauma over time from motions including grasping and ulnar deviation may lead to this condition, which is more common in women than men.[9] Repetitive trauma leads to noninflammatory thickening of the fibrous sheath surrounding the first dorsal

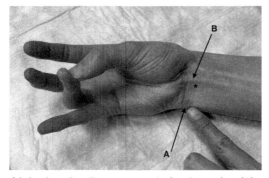

Fig. 2. Carpal tunnel injection site. Extensor carpi ulnaris tendon (A) and palmaris longus tendon (B); injection insertion site (*).

compartment of the hand. This thickening causes restriction in the gliding motion of the tendons contained within the sheath.[9] The first dorsal compartment contains the tendons that assist with thumb extension and abduction. It is most commonly diagnosed clinically using history of pain with repetitive thumb motion, particularly abduction and extension and a consistent examination. Physical examination findings that help to confirm de Quervain tenosynovitis include thickening and tenderness distal to the radial styloid as well as the Finkelstein test.[8] Patients who fail conservative treatment with antiinflammatories, activity modification, therapy, and bracing may be candidates for first dorsal compartment injection.

Anatomy: There are 6 dorsal compartments of the hand. The first dorsal compartment is affected by de Quervain tenosynovitis. This compartment contains the extensor pollicis brevis tendon, which allows for thumb extension, and the abductor pollicis longus, which allows for thumb abduction and extension. Placing the thumb in an abducted and extended position can help identify these tendons (**Fig. 3**). The first dorsal compartment makes up the anterior border of the anatomic snuffbox with the posterior border being the extensor pollicis longus tendon.

Preparation and Positioning

1. Gather the recommended supplies: cleansing solution, 0.5 to 1.5 inch, 25- to 27-gauge needle, 5 mL syringe, injectate, gauze, adhesive bandage, sterile skin marker.
2. Patient may be seated in front of a table or lying supine on an examination table. Place the ulnar aspect of the wrist on the table so that the affected radial aspect of the wrist faces upward.
3. A small towel roll can be used as needed to place the wrist further into ulnar deviation.
4. Prepare syringe with 0.5 to 1 mL of anesthetic and 0.5 mL of corticosteroid. Dexamethasone is preferred for this superficial injection site to minimize risk for skin atrophy and discoloration.

Procedure

1. Identify the abductor pollicis longus and extensor pollicis brevis at the level of the radial styloid of the wrist (see **Fig. 3**).
2. Identify the space between these 2 tendons. Use a skin marker to identify the injection site.
3. The injection site should be cleaned with appropriate antiseptic solution.
4. Insert needle into marked site parallel to the tendons in a distal to proximal approach at a 30-degree angle.

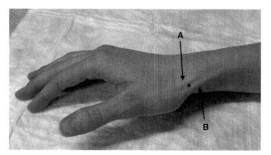

Fig. 3. First dorsal compartment injection site. Extensor pollicis brevis (A) and abductor pollicis longus (B) and at the level of the radial styloid of the wrist, injection site (*).

5. When the needle is inserted approximately $1/4$ inch, aspirate to ensure no return of blood.
6. Slowly push solution into the first dorsal compartment space. If resistance is felt, slightly withdraw and redirect the needle angle to avoid intratendinous injection.
7. Remove needle and clean site with gauze. Apply adhesive bandage.
8. Provide postprocedure care and reassess pain.

FLEXOR TENDON SHEATH

Diagnosis: Trigger finger, also known as digital flexor tenosynovitis, is a common cause of finger pain and dysfunction. Patients will classically present with an initial complaint of painless locking or catching of the affected finger,[10] and this may progress to have a tender palpable nodule overlying the palmar aspect of the metacarpophalangeal (MCP) as well as loss of flexion or extension of the finger. Risk factors for development include repetitive use activities, diabetes, rheumatoid arthritis, female gender, and fifth or sixth decade of life.[6] This condition is likely due to inflammation and swelling, resulting in either the flexor tendon or the pulley itself becoming too thick at the level where the tendons must pass through the pulley.[8,10] Injection can be helpful for alleviating symptoms or pain, catching, or locking of the affected finger.

Anatomy: The flexor surface of each finger has a series of fibrous sheaths known as pulleys that assist with the finger's ability to maximize its strength and efficiency with flexion. There are 5 annular pulleys (A1–A5) as well as 3 cruciform pulleys (C1–C3) and the palmar aponeurosis. The A1 pulley, which is most proximal, is the fibrous sheath most commonly associated with trigger finger and is located at the distal palmar crease.[11] The flexor digitorum longus and flexor digitorum superficialis tendons glide underneath the annular pulleys.

Preparation and Positioning

1. Gather the recommended supplies: cleansing solution, 0.5 to 1.5 inch 25- to 27-gauge needle, 5 mL syringe, injectate, gauze, adhesive bandage, sterile skin marker.
2. Patient may be seated in front of a table or lying supine on an examination table.
3. Place hand supine on the table with all fingers resting comfortably in an extended position.
4. Prepare syringe with 0.5 mL of anesthetic and 0.5 mL of corticosteroid. Dexamethasone is preferred for this superficial injection site to minimize risk for skin atrophy and discoloration.

Procedure

1. Identify the distal palmar crease just proximal to the MCP of the affected hand and mark the midline with a skin marker to assist with avoiding the neurovascular bundles lateral to the tendon (**Fig. 4**).
2. The injection site should be cleaned with appropriate antiseptic solution.
3. Insert the needle bevel up into marked site parallel to the tendons in a proximal to distal approach, toward the fingertips, at a 30-degree angle stopping superficial to the tendon.
4. Aspirate to ensure there is no blood.
5. Ask the patient to flex and extend the affected digit to assist in determining if the needle is intratendinous. The needle will move with flexion and extension if intratendinous, which should prompt slight withdrawal before injection.

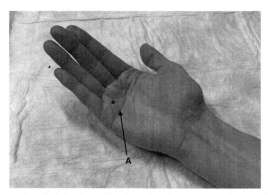

Fig. 4. Flexor tendon sheath injection site. Distal palmar crease (A) and injection site (*).

6. Slowly push solution into the space. To avoid intratendinous injection, if met with resistance, slightly withdraw the needle slightly, repeat aspiration, and attempt again to inject.
7. Remove needle and clean site with gauze. Apply adhesive bandage.
8. Provide postprocedure care and reassess pain.

PLANTAR FASCIA

<u>Diagnosis</u>: plantar fasciitis is a common condition of the fascia supporting the arch of the foot. It is often a chronic tendinopathy and less often inflammatory. The injured fascia stems from repetitive microtrauma through stress, overuse, or injury. Symptoms typically include pain that is worse in the morning and with prolonged standing but improves with continued activity. Risk factors for planta fasciitis include improper footwear, overuse, pes planus or cavus deformity, weak intrinsic foot musculature, decreased dorsiflexion, elevated body mass index, and sedentary lifestyle. Mainstay of therapy includes the use of stretching and strengthening routines with a focus on gastrocnemius and pedal muscles. Patients who fail conservative treatment with anti-inflammatories, activity modification, appropriate shoe wear, and therapy may be candidates for injection.

<u>Anatomy</u>: the plantar fascia is located just superior to the calcaneal fat pad, starting at the medial tuberosity of the calcaneus and extending distally to insert at the metatarsals. Care should be taken to avoid injection of the fat pad, as it can lead to atrophy and necrosis, further increasing pain. Fascial rupture occurs in approximately 2.4% of patients receiving corticosteroid injections, and patients undergoing injection should be counseled regarding this risk.[8] It should be noted that ultrasound-guided injection, which allows for better visualization of this anatomy, is becoming more prominent and has been shown to be more accurate and provide superior clinical outcomes.

Preparation and Positioning

1. Gather recommended supplies: cleansing solution, 1 to 1.5 inch, 25- to 27-gauge needle, 5 mL syringe, injectate, gauze, adhesive bandage, sterile skin marker.
2. Prepare syringe with desired corticosteroid and 3 mL of anesthetic.
3. Position the patient supine with their leg outstretched on and supported by the table. The foot should be relaxed in this position, with the medial aspect of the affected foot facing you.
4. The ideal approach is to inject medially.

Procedure

1. Locate the point of maximal tenderness through palpation and mark with a skin marker.
2. The injection site should be cleaned with appropriate antiseptic solution.
3. Insert needle at point of maximal tenderness, ensuring the needle is parallel to and 1 to 2 cm cephalad the sole of the foot, just caudal to the calcaneus, and distal to the fascial insertion.
4. Inject the solution throughout the space by gently fanning the needle under the fascia. Do not push against resistance. Gently draw back from the space as the solution completes, taking care not to divert into the fat pad.
5. Remove needle and clean site with gauze. Apply adhesive bandage.
6. When hemostasis is achieved the patient can gently flex and extend their affected foot to move the steroid throughout the subfascial plane.
7. Provide postprocedure care and reassess pain.

GANGLION CYST

Diagnosis: ganglion cysts are thick, rubbery cystic fluid–filled sacs located underneath the skin, often found at the wrist.[11,12] These cysts are often painless but can compress local tissue and nerves or prove to be aesthetically displeasing. Indications for aspiration and injection include impairment of wrist function, rapid growth, pain, or sensory change. Cysts can be aspirated, followed by a steroid injection to reduce inflammation and decrease chances of the cyst recurrence. Cysts recur approximately 50% of the time after aspiration and injection.

Anatomy: ganglion cysts are most frequently located on the dorsal side of the wrist above tendon sheaths and fascia. Proximity to the neurovascular structures should be noted before injection (**Fig. 5**).

Preparation and Positioning

1. Gather recommended supplies: cleansing solution, 1 to 1.5 inch 25-gauge needle, 18-gauge needle, 3 mL syringes, 20 to 25 mL syringe, injectate, hemostat, gauze, adhesive bandage, and sterile skin marker.
2. Prepare a 3 mL syringe with 1 to 2 mL of the local anesthetic with a 25-gauge needle for anesthesia. An 18-gauge needle on a 10 to 20 mL syringe should be set aside for the aspiration.
3. If steroid injection is planned after aspiration prepare a separate syringe. We recommend 0.5 mL dexamethasone or triamcinolone mixed with 0.5 mL of 1% lidocaine.[12,13]
4. Have the patient rest their wrist in a comfortable position with the cyst easily accessible.

Procedure

1. Locate local vasculature (radial or ulnar artery) to avoid during the procedure.
2. Locate the borders of the ganglion cyst, marking it with skin marker.
3. The injection site should be cleaned with appropriate antiseptic solution.
4. Inject lidocaine solution subcutaneously to create a wheal where the aspiration needle will be inserted. Withdraw lidocaine needle and allow 1 to 2 minutes for effect.
5. Insert the 18-gauge aspiration needle through the wheal into the cyst and apply slow constant pressure on the syringe to aspirate the thick jellylike liquid.

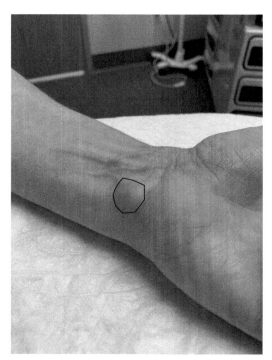

Fig. 5. Ganglion cyst encircled.

6. If after aspiration, steroid injection is planned, the 18-gauge needle can be held in place with a hemostat, whereas the syringe containing steroid is attached and subsequently inject into the cyst.
7. Remove needle and clean site with gauze. Apply adhesive bandage. Consider compression dressing to help prevent fluid from reaccumulating.
8. Provide postprocedure care and reassess pain.

TRIGGER POINT

Diagnosis: trigger points are hard nodules palpated at defined locations in muscles, differentiated from tender points in that they cause regional pain that does not follow dermatome patterns. Frequently they cause latent pain that may not be pronounced until pressure is placed directly over the nodule. Indications for injection include clustering of trigger points causing myofascial pain syndrome and treatment of recurring pain due to the trigger points.[14]

Anatomy: trigger points can occur in muscles throughout the body but are primarily focused in the neck and shoulder region[15] (**Fig. 6**). Nodules can be palpated through the overlying tissue and are usually within 0.5 to 1.5 inches of the surface, although body habitus may cause this to differ.

Preparation and Positioning

1. Gather recommended supplies: cleansing solution, 0.5 to 1.5 inch 22- to 25-gauge needle, 1 to 5 mL syringe, injectate, gauze, adhesive bandage, sterile skin marker.
2. Positioning of the patient will depend on the location of the injection but should allow for ease of access to the injection site, stability of the patient, and proper control of the needle by the physician.

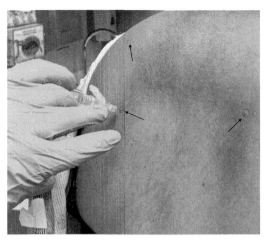

Fig. 6. Trigger point injection, arrows highlighting prepped injection sites.

3. Prepare syringe with 1 to 2 mL anesthetic with 22- to 25-gauge needle.
4. If performing a lidocaine and steroid injection, mix 1 to 2 mL of steroid with anesthetic in one 5 mL syringe for injection.

Procedural Approach

1. Palpate the nodule and press down to fix it between 2 fingers, so that it does not move during the procedure, and mark the site of the nodule with a marking pen.
2. The injection site should be cleaned with appropriate antiseptic solution.
3. Firmly hold the nodule with fingers on either side and insert the needle into nodule at a 90° angle to the skin. The muscle may twitch once needle has entered trigger point.
4. Aspirate to ensure no blood return.
5. Inject solution while slowly withdrawing needle, taking care to inject laterally, inferiorly, and superiorly.
6. Alternately, one can use a Z-track injection method.
   ○ Pull the skin above marked site taut upward with stabilizing hand. Insert needle at marked site at 45-degree angle from skin.
   ○ Insert needle completely into the musculature, and as you slowly withdraw and dispense solution, release the skin and pull taut again repeatedly to allow "Z track" of solution release throughout the affected site.
7. Remove needle and clean site with gauze. Apply pressure with gauze for 2 minutes after needle fully removed to prevent hematoma.
8. Apply adhesive bandage and have patient actively move affected muscle through full range of motion. Improvement in pain should be immediate.
9. Provide postprocedure care and reassess pain.

SUMMARY

Small joint, tendon, and myofascial injections offer the opportunity to provide pain relief and antiinflammatory benefit when first-line conservative treatment fails. Patients should be educated on the risks of injection before an informed decision to proceed can be made. The provider should have a strong understanding of indications, contraindications, and the local anatomy and landmarks at the site of injection. If there is uncertainty regarding indications, potential contraindications, anatomy, or technique for injection, referral to a sports medicine or orthopedic specialist is recommended.

CLINICS CARE POINTS

- Injections and aspirations are used for both diagnostic and therapeutic purposes.
- Indications, contraindications, and risks of the procedure should be addressed during the informed consent process.
- To avoid intratendinous injection at any site, if met with resistance, withdraw the needle slightly, repeat aspiration, and attempt again to inject.
- Injectable anesthetics will be effective typically within seconds to minutes and duration varies with short-acting (3–4 hours) and long-acting (6–8 hours) options.
- Injectable steroids vary in their time to onset, but most of the patients have symptom relief within weeks with average effects lasting 3 months.

DISCLOSURE

The authors have nothing to disclose.

REFERENCES

1. Lutrzykowski CJ, OConnor FG, Barkdull T. Common injections in sports medicine: general principles and specific techniques. In: O'Connor FG, editor. Acsm's sports medicine: a comprehensive review. Philadelphia (PA): Wolters Kluwer Health/Lippincott Williams & Wilkins; 2013. p. 520–7.
2. Pytiak AV, Viddal AF, Wolcot M. Injections in the athlete. In: Madden CC, Netter FH, editors. Netter's sports medicine. Philadelphia (PA): Saunders/Elsevier; 2010. p. 499–505.
3. McNabb JW, Ovid Technologies I. A practical guide to joint & soft tissue injection & aspiration: an illustrated text for primary care providers. 2nd edition. Philadelphia (PA): Wolters Kluwer Health/Lippincott Williams & Wilkins; 2010. p. 1–5.
4. Rai K, Sylvester J. Musculoskeletal Injections. Curr Sports Med Rep 2020;19(6): 191–3.
5. Honchurak E, Monica J. Complications associated with intra-articular and extra-articular corticosteroid injection. J Bone Joint Surg 2016;4(12):e2.
6. Urits I, Smoots D, Anantuni L, et al. Injection techniques for common chronic pain conditions of the hand: a comprehensive review. Pain Ther 2020;9(1):129–42.
7. Padua A, Coraci D, Erra C, et al. Carpal tunnel syndrome: clinical features, diagnosis, and management. Lancet Neurol 2016;15(12):1273–84.
8. Tallia AF, Cardone DA. Diagnostic and therapeutic injection of the wrist and hand region. Am Fam Physician 2003;67(4):745–50.
9. Ilyas AM, Ast M, Schaffer AA, et al. De quervain tenosynovitis of the wrist. J Am Acad Orthop Surg 2007;15(12):757–64.
10. Makkouk AH, Oetgen ME, Swigart CR, et al. Trigger finger: etiology, evaluation, and treatment. Curr Rev Musculoskelet Med 2008;1(2):92–6.
11. Goff JD, Crawford R. Diagnosis and treatment of plantar fasciitis. Am Fam Physician 2011;84(6):676–82.
12. Lim AT, How CH, Tan B. Management of plantar fasciitis in the outpatient setting. Singapore Med J 2016;57(4):168–71.

13. Doug Aukerman, M. F. (2009). Plantar Fascia Injection. In: E.J. Mayeaux Jr, editor. Essential guide to primary care procedures (pp. 828-833). Philadelphia, PA: Wolters Kluwer.

14. Boyd, A., & Wissink, S. (2009). Wrist Ganglia Aspiration and Injection. In: E.J. Mayeaux Jr, editor. Essential guide to primary care procedures (pp. 904-908). Philadelphia, PA: Wolters Kluwer.

15. EJ. Mayeaux Jr (2009). Trigger Point Injection. In E.J. Mayeaux Jr, editor. Essential guide to primary care procedure (pp. 898 - 902). Philadelphia, PA: Wolters Kluwer.

Managing Fractures and Sprains

Nathan Falk, MD, MBA[a],*, Bernadette Pendergraph, MD[b,1], T. Jason Meredith, MD[c], George Le, MD[b,1], Hannah Hornsby, MD[d]

KEYWORDS

- Fracture • Sprain • Splint • Cast • Metacarpal • Malleolus • Upper extremity
- Lower extremity

KEY POINTS

- After appropriate imaging and fracture diagnosis, immobilization and determination of definitive management, either nonoperative or operative, is critical. After initial stabilization, complicated fractures should be referred to a specialist.
- Appropriate immobilization is imperative to injury healing.
- In general, short-term immobilization of the shoulder and the elbow decreases the future stiffness of these joints, often achieved with simple slings or short-term splinting.
- Posterior splints are appropriate for the acute treatment of metatarsal shaft fractures, Jones fractures, and nondisplaced malleolar fractures.
- Controlled ankle movement walker boots are used for second to fifth metatarsal shaft fractures, zone 1 fractures of the proximal fifth metatarsal fractures, great toe fractures, and nonoperative ankle fractures.

 Video content accompanies this article at http://www.primarycare.theclinics. com.

INTRODUCTION

Primary care physicians are often the first to evaluate patients with extremity injuries. Identification of fractures and sprains and their proper management is paramount. The annual incidence of fractures is 3.6%, with upper extremity fractures accounting for roughly half of those injuries.[1] All injuries should include a neurovascular examination.

[a] Florida State University, 1201 1st Street South, Suite 100A, Winter Haven, FL 33880, USA; [b] Harbor-UCLA Medical Center, Torrance, CA, USA; [c] Department of Family Medicine, UNMC Family Medicine Residency Program, University of Nebraska Medical Center College of Medicine, 983075 Nebraska Medical Center, Omaha, NE 68198-3075, USA; [d] Department of Family Medicine, Offutt AFB/UNMC Family Medicine Residency Program, University of Nebraska Medical Center College of Medicine, 983075 Nebraska Medical Center, Omaha, NE 68198-3075, USA
[1] Present address: 1403 W Lomita Boulevard 2nd Floor, Harbor City, CA 90710.
* Corresponding author.
E-mail address: nfalk@fsu.edu

Prim Care Clin Office Pract 49 (2022) 145–161
https://doi.org/10.1016/j.pop.2021.10.007
0095-4543/22/© 2021 Elsevier Inc. All rights reserved.

primarycare.theclinics.com

After appropriate imaging is obtained, immobilization and determination of definitive management, either nonoperative or operative, is critical. Appropriate immobilization is imperative to promote injury healing. In general, short-term immobilization of the shoulder and the elbow decreases the future stiffness of these joints, often achieved with simple slings or short-term splinting.[2,3] Gutter splints are often used for phalanx or metacarpal fractures (**Fig. 1**). Carpal bone and distal radius fractures usually require short-term volar splinting with definitive treatment to follow, most often with a short-arm cast if nonoperative treatment is deemed appropriate.[4,5]

Posterior splints are appropriate for the acute treatment of metatarsal shaft fractures, Jones fractures, and nondisplaced malleolar fractures and should extend from the plantar surface of the great toe to about 2 inches distal to the fibular head (**Fig. 2**).[4,6] Controlled ankle movement (CAM) boots are used for second to fifth metatarsal shaft fractures, zone 1 fractures of the proximal fifth metatarsal fractures, great toe fractures, and nonoperative ankle fractures (**Fig. 3**).[7] Nondisplaced or minimally displaced lesser toe fractures may be managed with buddy taping and a hard-soled shoe.

SHOULDER

Acromioclavicular (AC) joint injuries are common, accounting for 9% to 12% of shoulder injuries. They often result from a fall onto the shoulder with the arm adducted. The injury is graded based on the displacement of the clavicle superiorly, medially, or posteriorly. Grades 1 and 2, with less than 25% elevation of the clavicle, are treated in a sling for comfort for 1 to 2 weeks, followed by range of motion.[2] All other AC sprains may need surgical intervention. The brachial plexus should be evaluated for injury.

The glenohumeral joint is the most dislocated joint resulting from a combination of abduction, external rotation, and extension forces to the joint.[2] Injury to the axillary nerve is evaluated by checking lateral shoulder sensation and action of the deltoid muscle. Rotator cuff injuries are common with advancing age. In an uncomplicated dislocation, the shoulder is reduced, and a sling is used for 1 to 2 weeks, followed by range of motion and progressive strengthening.[2]

Clavicle fractures account for 3% of all fractures and commonly occur from a fall on the top of the shoulder or an axial load through the clavicle.[2] These injuries can be

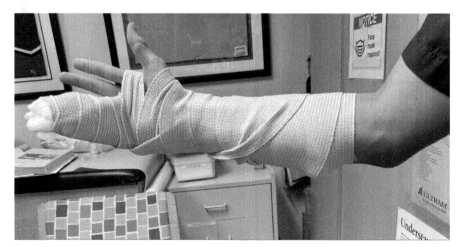

Fig. 1. Ulnar gutter splint.

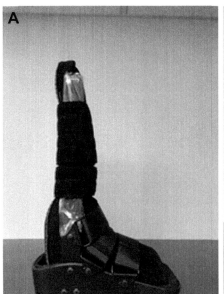 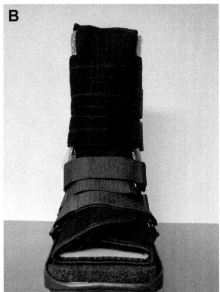

Fig. 2. (*A, B*) CAM boot.

open or the skin can be tented and may rarely be associated with injuries to the great vessels, lungs, and brachial plexus. Medial and middle third fractures that are not displaced more than 100% of bone width or shortened more than 2 cm can be treated with a sling for 3 weeks, followed by range of motion exercises. Distal third fractures with displacement should prompt surgical evaluation.[8]

Proximal humerus fractures account for 5% of all fractures.[9] Because many proximal humerus fractures are fragility fractures, they are more common in the elderly and women and are often associated with distal radius and femur fractures.[1] Proximal humerus fractures can be evaluated by the Neer classification.[6] These fractures are considered displaced if angulated more than 45° or displaced by greater than 1 cm.[1] If the fracture is stable and nondisplaced, it can be managed with a sling for 2 weeks (up to 4–6 weeks for comfort), followed by early physical therapy with passive range of motion within a few days of the original injury. For fractures with angulation less than 45°, the collar with cuff sling is preferred for stabilization.[1,9,10] Displaced fractures require surgical management.

HUMERAL SHAFT

Humeral shaft fractures account for 5% of fractures and are seen more in elderly patients.[9,11] Humeral shaft fractures are classified by the AO classification paying attention to type (simple, wedge, complex) and pattern (spiral, oblique, transverse). Many humeral shaft fractures are minimally displaced, and management is nonsurgical.[12] Minimally displaced criteria include less than 3 cm of shortening, 15° of rotation, 20° of anterior bowing, and 30° of varus or valgus angulation. Patients can be managed with a hanging cast or coaptation splint for 1 to 2 weeks, followed by functional bracing for at least 8 weeks from initial injury (**Fig. 4**, Video 1).[12] Because of the location of these fractures, injury to the radial nerve must also be evaluated.[1,9]

Distal humerus fractures account for 2% of total fractures and are seen in all age groups.[1] They are classified by the AO classification and can occur as supracondylar,

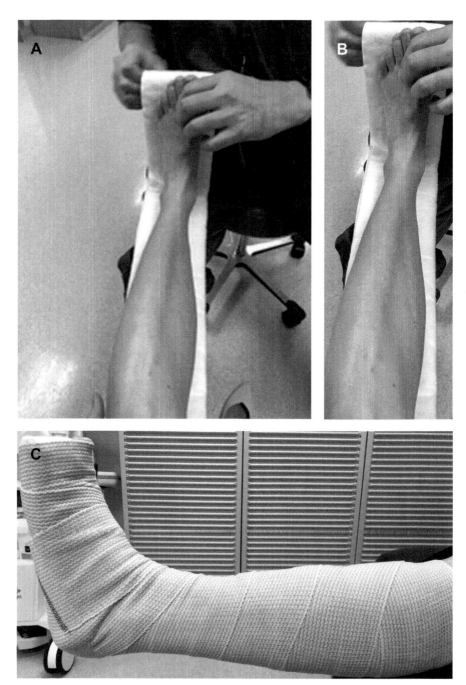

Figs. 3. (*A–C*) Short-leg posterior splint.

transcondylar, intercondylar, and epicondylar.[1] When assessing whether nonoperative management is an option, one must evaluate for the absence of injuries to the brachial artery and nerves (radial, median, and ulnar). Nondisplaced supracondylar

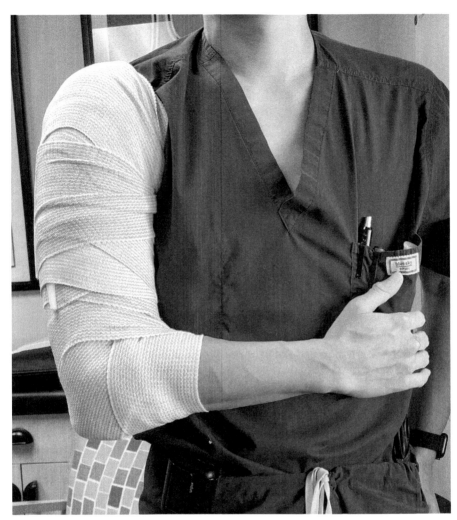

Fig. 4. Coaptation splint.

fractures can be managed with a posterior long arm splint or cast with the elbow flexed to at least 90° for 2 to 3 weeks, followed by progressive range of motion in a hinged brace.[1] Close follow-up (within 1 week) is recommended to monitor for displacement.[1] Fractures that are displaced or have an intraarticular component should have surgical evaluation.[9]

ELBOW

Olecranon fractures are seen in all ages resulting from direct trauma. During evaluation, one must assess for ulnar nerve injury. These fractures usually need surgical evaluation. If the fracture is nondisplaced, stable at 90° of flexion, and has an intact extensor mechanism, nonoperative management in a long arm cast for 3 weeks with the elbow flexed to 90° is recommended (**Fig. 5**, Video 2).[13] Follow-up radiographs should be performed within 1 week to assess fracture healing and alignment.

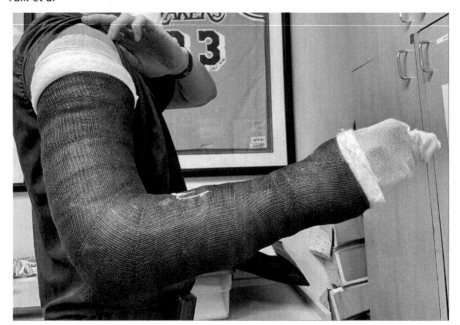

Fig. 5. Long arm cast.

Radial head fractures can occur from a fall onto an outstretched hand. Nondisplaced or minimally displaced radial head fractures can be treated nonoperatively with a pressure bandage and sling. Early mobilization should begin as soon as possible.[3]

FOREARM

Forearm fractures are less common than other upper extremity fractures but occur from axial load or direct trauma.[1] Evaluation for injuries to neurovascular structures, the joints proximal and distal to the injury (the distal radial ulnar joint [DRUJ] and elbow), and compartment syndrome are required to assess whether nonoperative management is an option. Fractures that involve dislocations (Monteggia and Galeazzi) are managed surgically.[1]

Isolated, stable, and nondisplaced radius fractures can be managed nonoperatively with a long arm cast, with the elbow in 90° of flexion with a neutral wrist in a slightly extended position. The cast should start from the distal palmar crease and extend proximally to the midhumerus.[4]

Nightstick fractures are named for isolated ulna fractures resulting from the force of a policeman's nightstick onto the arm. Unstable/open fractures, displacement greater than 50%, and angulation more than 15° need surgical evaluation. Otherwise, nondisplaced ulna fractures are treated nonoperatively with a sugar-tong splint for 1 week, followed by functional bracing and early mobilization (**Fig. 6**, Video 3).[4,14] When casted, isolated ulnar fractures have a relatively high risk of nonunion, so close follow-up is recommended.[1]

DISTAL RADIUS

Distal radius fractures are the most common fractures in older adults and are usually due to a fall.[1] The most common type of distal radius fracture is Colles, where there is dorsal displacement followed by Smith fracture with volar displacement.[1]

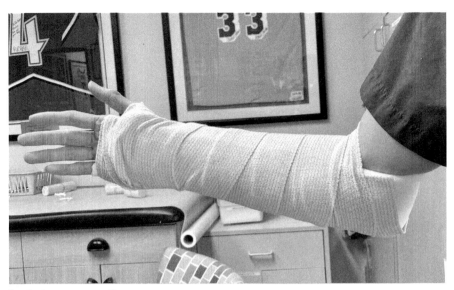

Fig. 6. Sugar tong splint.

Nondisplaced and stable fractures can be managed initially with a sugar tong splint followed by short arm cast.[4] The sugar tong splint should start from the proximal palmar crease, with the forearm in neutral position. The splint will wrap around the elbow and up the forearm's dorsal surface up to the metacarpophalangeal (MCP) joints, where the wrist should be in a slightly extended position. The short arm cast should start from the distal palmar crease and extend to the forearm's proximal third (see Video 2). The wrist should be in a neutral position and slightly extended. For buckle fractures more commonly encountered in pediatric patients, a volar arm splint is preferable to a short arm cast.[4]

CARPALS

Wrist sprains are common and occur acutely from a fall onto an outstretched hand or chronically from repetitive motions. The most common ligaments sprained are the scapholunate ligament and the triangular fibrocartilage complex.[15] If radiographs do not show disruption to the carpal row alignment and the DRUJ is intact, a wrist splint or short arm cast can be used for immobilization. If carpal row disruption is present, orthopedic consultation is recommended.

Carpal fractures make up approximately 20% of all hand and wrist fractures, with scaphoid accounting for most of them.[16,17] Consideration for referral should be given for most carpal bone fractures. A thumb spica cast is used to stabilize nondisplaced, stable trapezium, trapezoid, lunate, and capitate fractures. A thumb spica cast should cover the interphalangeal joint of the first metacarpal and extend up to the proximal third of the forearm. **Fig. 7** and Video 2 demonstrate a long-arm thumb spica cast; however, please note that a short-arm thumb spica cast is reasonable for trapezium fractures. The wrist should be in 25° of extension with the thumb in a "position of function."[4]

Scaphoid fractures usually result from an axial impact with a hyperextended wrist, seen with a fall onto an outstretched hand. Most scaphoid fractures occur at the waist.[16] A long arm thumb spica (see **Fig. 7**, see Video 2) cast for 6 weeks can be

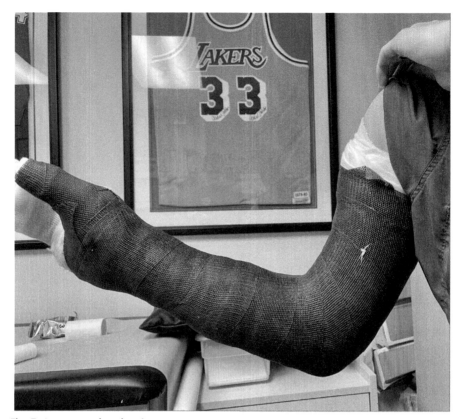

Fig. 7. Long arm thumb spica cast.

used if the scaphoid fracture is to the distal pole or scaphoid waist, acute, stable, non-displaced (less than 1 mm), noncomminuted, and at acceptable angles (scapholunate less than 60° and intrascaphoid <35°).[18] The long arm thumb spica cast should control wrist extension and ulnar deviation to stabilize the fracture. After 6 weeks, the long arm thumb spica cast should be replaced with a short arm thumb spica cast until the fracture is fully healed.[19]

Expected time for the full union of a scaphoid fracture depends on location, up to 6 weeks for the distal scaphoid and more than 10 weeks for the proximal scaphoid.[18] Referral to a hand surgeon is recommended for proximal scaphoid fractures (and consideration of referral for distal and waist fractures), as there are risks of long-term complications from avascular necrosis and nonunion. If the scaphoid injury is suspected, but the initial radiographs are abnormal, a thumb spica splint should be used with follow-up imaging in 7 to 10 days.[17]

After the scaphoid, the triquetrum is the most common carpal fracture.[17] Triquetrum fractures can be managed with a short arm cast. They can, along with pisiform fractures, also be managed with an ulnar gutter splint.[4,17]

A hook of hamate fracture can be managed with a modified thumb spica cast that has the wrist positioned in slight flexion and immobilizes fourth and fifth MCP joints in maximum flexion. The body of the hamate fracture can be managed with a volar short arm splint with the hand in a position of function.[17]

METACARPAL

Metacarpal fractures are classified according to location of the fracture (eg, the metacarpal head, neck, shaft, and base).[20] Unstable and intraarticular metacarpal fractures (step off greater than 1 mm or >25% of articular surface) and fractures involving the head or base should be referred to a hand specialist. Stable, nonrotated metacarpal neck fractures have greater acceptable fracture angulation. For factures to the second and third metacarpal neck, less than 10 to 15° of angulation is acceptable. For the fourth and fifth metacarpal neck fractures, less than 30° and 40° of angulation, respectively, is acceptable.[20]

The most common metacarpal fracture is the fifth metacarpal neck fracture (frequently referred to as a "boxer fracture").[17] The mechanism of injury involves punching an object. Stable, nondisplaced, nonrotated, and tolerable angulated fractures of the fourth and fifth metacarpal neck can be managed in an ulnar gutter splint, with buddy taping for 4 weeks.[20] The splint should cover the distal interphalangeal (DIP) joint and extend proximally past the mid-forearm. The wrist should be in slight extension, with the MCP joints flexed at 70 to 90° and the proximal interphalangeal (PIP) and DIP joints flexed at 5 to 10° (see **Fig. 1**).[4] A radial gutter splint is used for the immobilization of second and third metacarpal neck fractures.

Stable, nondisplaced, nonrotated metacarpal shaft fractures can be reduced and managed with a gutter splint or cast (radial gutter for second and third metacarpal and ulnar gutter for fourth and fifth metacarpal) (Videos 4 and 5).[17,20] The splint should cover the DIP joint of the second and third metacarpal and extend proximally past the mid-forearm. The wrist should be placed in slight extension, the MCP joints flexed at 70 to 90° and the proximal interphalangeal and distal interphalangeal joints flexed at 5 to 10°.[4] Surgical evaluation should be obtained if the fracture involves any rotational deformities, greater than 10° of dorsal angulation (for second and third metacarpals) or greater than 20° and 30° of dorsal angulation (for fourth and fifth metacarpals, respectively).[20]

Fractures of the first metacarpal include the Bennett and Rolando fractures. Acute management of these fractures involve using a thumb spica splint. These fractures should be referred to a hand specialist for further management.[17]

First metacarpal joint collateral ligament sprains, such as gamekeeper's or skier's thumb (insufficiency of the ulnar collateral ligament), can be managed with a thumb spica splint for 4 to 6 weeks. Tears of the collateral ligament require surgical evaluation.[21]

PHALANX

Volar lip fracture of the base of the middle phalanx is caused by dorsal PIP fracture-dislocation. If the fracture involves greater than 30% of the intraarticular surface and is displaced or unstable, referral to a hand specialist is indicated. Small avulsions of the volar lip may be managed with buddy taping for 6 weeks. Otherwise, this fracture can be managed with a 20° dorsal extension block splint with buddy taping for 2 weeks, followed by decreasing flexion by 10° after each week. After close follow-up and radiographic evidence that reduction is maintained and stable, the splint can be removed, but buddy taping should continue for at least 3 more weeks.[22,23]

Dorsal lip fracture of the base of the middle phalanx, caused by volar PIP fracture-dislocation, can cause boutonniere deformities. If the fracture involves less than 30% to 40% of the intraarticular surface or there is less than 2 mm of displacement, it can be managed with a dorsal splint with full PIP extension and buddy taping for 4 to 6 weeks, followed by dynamic extension splint for 2 more weeks.[17,22,23]

Proximal and middle phalangeal extraarticular fractures that are stable, nondisplaced, and nonangulated can be managed with a dorsal or gutter splint with full PIP extension, wrist in 30° of extension, MCP in 90° of flexion, and buddy taping for 6 weeks.[16,23]

Distal phalanx (Tuft) fractures occur from crush injuries. If the fracture remains stable and extraarticular, it should be wrapped with an aluminum splint with the DIP joint in extension.[4,17,22]

Mallet finger, where the distal phalanx remains in unopposed flexion due to the avulsion of the extensor digitorum tendon from the dorsal base of the distal phalanx, is seen in a jam injury (such as when a ball or other object strikes the tip of the phalanx, resulting in a forced bending of the DIP joint). The distal phalanx should be continuously splinted in slight hyperextension for 6 to 8 weeks.[4,17,22]

Jersey finger, named for injuries caused by grabbing an opponent's jersey, occurs when the distal phalanx remains in unopposed extension due to the avulsion of the flexor digitorum profundus from the volar base of the distal phalanx. Surgical evaluation is indicated.[17,22]

KNEE
Medial Collateral Ligament Injuries

Injury usually occurs during sport when a valgus force is applied to a planted knee and described as the knee "giving way" and "popping." Physical examination will show medial opening with valgus stress and tenderness to palpation over the medial aspect of the knee. Valgus and varus testing for collateral ligament injuries should occur with the knee flexed to 30° and in full extension. Joint space gapping at full extension is concerning for associated cruciate injury within the knee. With grade 1 injuries, only a small amount of MCL fibers are compromised leading to minimal gapping on valgus testing. Grade 2 injuries involve more fibers creating more laxity on valgus testing but with an end point still present. Grade 3 injuries are a complete tear of the MCL, leading to gross joint instability and no end point on valgus testing.

Grade 1 and 2 injuries are managed with early rehab and range of motion. Use of a hinged knee brace can help prevent further valgus injury and provide patients a sense of increased knee stability. Weight bearing as tolerated is appropriate. Grade 3 tears rarely happen in isolation and are usually associated with other internal derangements of the knee. Advanced imaging with MRI and orthopedic referral are advised. With appropriate rehabilitation, patients with grade 1 or 2 injuries often return to sport or work in a few weeks. Inappropriate knee immobilizer usage can lead to excessive joint stiffness and need for prolonged rehabilitation. Knee immobilizers have limited indications and should only be used after patellar tendon ruptures, MCL sprains, patellar fractures, or dislocations.[24]

Lateral Collateral Ligament Injuries

Lateral collateral ligament (LCL) injuries are uncommon.[25] When they do occur, they are usually associated with other soft tissue injuries including posterolateral corner injuries, cruciate ligament strain, and lateral meniscus injuries (these associated injuries will require orthopedic evaluation). Patients will endorse pain over the lateral joint line and a sensation of instability. Physical examination will demonstrate lateral opening with the application of varus stress. Grading of LCL tears is the same as MCL injuries.

Initial management for isolated injuries includes RICE (rest, ice, compression and elevation) and physical therapy for grade 1 and 2 injuries. If patients do not demonstrate improvement after 6 to 8 weeks of rehabilitation, MRI and/or referral to orthopedics should be considered. Grade 3 injuries should be referred to orthopedics.

Patellar Fractures

Patellar fractures usually result from a direct force such as a dashboard injury or fall.[26] Physical examination will reveal a rapidly developed effusion and tenderness to palpation. Obtain standard anteroposterior (AP) and lateral knee plain film radiographs. Patellar fracture patterns include stellate, comminuted, transverse, or vertical. Displacement is defined by step-off greater than 2 to 3 mm and fracture gap greater than 1 to 4 mm.[26]

Primary care physicians should only manage vertical, nondisplaced patellar fractures; all other injury types require an orthopedics referral.[5,26] Conservative management involves initial non–weight bearing status in a knee immobilizer for 5 to 7 days with transition to a removable hinged knee brace locked in extension.[5] Patient should remain non–weight bearing and begin straight leg raises while in the brace. Plain film radiographs should be repeated at 2 weeks to assess fracture alignment and subsequently at 4 to 6 weeks to document healing/union.[5] Patellar fractures can take up to 8 to 10 weeks to demonstrate radiographic healing. After radiographic evidence of healing, the brace can be removed and physical therapy initiated.

TIBIA
Toddler Fracture

This distinct type of tibial injury occurs in children between 9 months and 3 years of age, resulting in a spiral fracture of the middle or distal tibia. These fractures occur by a twisting injury while the child is falling, tripping, or stumbling.[27] Children will present with acute onset of limping or refusal to bear weight. Multiple views of the tibia should be obtained with plain films. Initial imaging can often be negative.

If a fracture is suspected but imaging is negative, treat appropriately and repeat imaging in 10 to 14 days.[28] Definitive management is a long leg cast for 3 weeks followed by 2 weeks in a short leg walking cast (SLWC) with weight bearing as tolerated. These fractures are commonly healed by 6 to 8 weeks.[5] An open fracture, presence of multiple fractures, displacement greater than 2 mm, or fracture shortening are indications for orthopedic referral.[28]

MALLEOLUS
Pediatric Malleollar Fractures

The distal tibial physis begins to close at around 12 years of age in women and 14 years of age in men. The physis fuses in the midportion and progresses medially and then laterally. Fractures will present with swelling and tenderness over the physis. A standard 3-view ankle plain film series should be obtained when boney tenderness of either malleolus is present (similar to adults).

The Salter-Harris classification system is the most widely used approach to describe physeal injuries.[29] Knowing this system is imperative to appropriately manage pediatric fractures.

Classification

Salter-Harris I: the fracture extends directly through the growth plate. This type of fracture is more common in young children.

Salter-Harris II: the fracture enters the plane of the physis and exits through the metaphysis, and this leaves a portion of the metaphysis attached to the epiphyseal fragment.

Salter-Harris III: the fracture enters in the plane of the physis but exits through the epiphysis, making it an intraarticular fracture.

Salter-Harris IV: the fracture extends from the articular surface through the epiphysis, growth plate, and metaphysis.

Salter-Harris V: these fractures are a result of a crush injury. No displacement occurs; however, the physis may be damaged.

Physeal injuries can lead to early growth plate closure. Primary care physicians should only manage nondisplaced Salter-Harris type 1 and 2 fractures; all other injuries should be referred to orthopedics. Patients awaiting surgical evaluation should be placed in a bulky compression dressing and kept non–weight bearing. Nondisplaced type 1 fractures can be treated with a CAM walker boot for 4 weeks (see **Fig. 2**). For nondisplaced type II fractures, patients should initially be immobilized in a long leg cast with the knee in 30° of flexion. After 3 weeks, the cast can be exchanged for an SLWC or CAM boot for an additional 3 to 4 weeks.[5] Repeat imaging at 6 and 12 months postinjury should be obtained to assess for early closure.[30]

Adult Malleolar Fractures

These common lower extremity injuries often occur from an inversion or eversion injury to the ankle. Patients will usually have tenderness to palpation over the malleolus and inability to bear weight. The Ottawa ankle and midfoot rules dictate when ankle or foot plain films are needed after an acute ankle injury. For patients who have tenderness over either malleolus, a plain film of the ankle is required for those who are unable to bear weight for 4 steps immediately after the injury and in the office/emergency department or demonstrate tenderness to palpation over the distal 6 cm of the posterior lateral malleolus or medial malleolus. If patients have midfoot pain, dedicated 3-view foot plain films are required if patients who are unable to bear weight for 4 steps, have tenderness to palpation over the base of the fifth metatarsal, or tenderness to palpation over the navicular bone.[31] In adult patients, the Ottawa ankle rules have exceptional sensitivity (99.4%) but lack in specificity (35.3%); in pediatric patients the sensitivity remains excellent (97.9%) but with a slightly worse specificity (21%).[32]

In the acute setting, the patient should be placed in a CAM boot or lower extremity splint (posterior splint vs stirrup splint) with the ankle in neutral position. The patient is referred to orthopedics for open fractures, bimalleolar fracturs, fractures with greater than 2 mm of displacement, or loss of joint congruity/stability on plain films.[5]

It is imperative to determine whether an ankle fracture is stable or unstable with appropriate plain films. Unstable ankles, even if without obvious, significant bony injury, require operative management. The definitive treatment of lateral malleolus fractures requires appropriately identifying the injury according to the Weber classification system. After fracture treatment, it is important to refer the patient to physical therapy for additional ankle strengthening and proprioception rehabilitation.

Weber A fractures are those where the fracture line is distal to the tibiotalar joint line.[33] These fractures can be treated with weight bearing as tolerated in a CAM boot for 4 to 6 weeks.

Weber B fractures have fracture lines that extend into or toward the joint line. These fractures are susceptible to joint instability from associated soft tissue injuries and often require operative management. Providers should initially review the mortise view. A widened mortise is a sign of joint instability that requires operative intervention.[33] If a widened mortise is not present, stress views should be obtained. If stress views are normal, conservative management can be completed with the patient placed in a CAM boot and made non–weight bearing for 3 to 4 weeks. At the follow-up visit repeat films should be obtained to assess for healing, and if pain allows, the patient may then be transitioned to weight bearing as tolerated in the CAM boot for an additional 3 to 4 weeks.

Weber C fractures are those with fracture lines proximal to the joint space. These fractures should be referred to an orthopedic provider.

For isolated medial malleolus or posterior malleolus fractures, great care should be undertaken to rule out other associated injuries. Injuries to the deltoid ligament can make nondisplaced medial malleolus injuries unstable. Initial management of these injuries involves splinting for the first 5 to 7 days. At follow-up, if the fracture is truly isolated, they may be treated definitively with weight bearing as tolerated in a CAM boot for 4 to 6 weeks.[5]

High Ankle Sprains

High ankle sprains (HAS) are characterized by the disruption of the tibiofibular syndesmosis. HAS occur when the foot is planted in a dorsiflexed position and is subjected to an external rotation force.[34] The patient will often present with an inability to bear weight and anterior ankle pain. Multiple special tests exist to assess for syndesmotic injuries. The external rotation test and the squeeze test both have high interobserver reliability.[34] The external rotation test is completed with the patient's knee flexed to 90°. The ankle is externally rotated while stabilizing the tibia. A positive test is pain within the ankle. The squeeze test is performed by compressing the lower leg at the level of the midtibia; pain at the ankle is a positive test for an HAS. Ankle plain films should be obtained to assess joint stability and identify any associated fractures; changes in the mortise views will identify an unstable joint that requires operative management.[34] Plain films of the proximal tibia/fibula should be obtained if the squeeze test elicits proximal lower leg pain. Maisonneuve fractures of the proximal fibula can occur with HAS. Ottawa ankle rules are not applied to HAS.

Classification

Grade I: only a partial tear of the anterior inferior tibiofibular ligament (AITFL). Plain films will be normal; the joint is stable.

Grade II: partial disruption of the interosseous ligaments and AITFL.

Grade III: complete disruption of all syndesmotic ligaments, with or without involvement of the deltoid ligament.

HAS require longer healing time than classic lateral ankle sprains. Appropriate treatment of HAS depends on accurate grading of the injury. Grade 2 or 3 injuries and any injury with associated fractures should be referred to orthopedics for evaluation.[34,35] Grade 1 injuries should be placed in a CAM boot and made non–weight bearing for 3 weeks. If pain has improved at follow-up, the patient can be evaluated on their ability to complete a single leg hop. If they are able to complete a single leg hop, transition the patient to a lace-up ankle brace and begin rehabilitation.[35] If the patient is unable to complete a single leg hop, immobilization should be continued for an additional week. If after this period the patient is still unable to complete the maneuver, the patient should be referred to orthopedics for further evaluation. If the patient is able to complete the hop, treat as outlined earlier.[34] Athletes may return to full participation when they have full range of motion and are able to perform sport-specific drills pain free.[34]

METATARSAL
Metatarsal Shaft Fractures

Shaft fractures often result from direct trauma. Ecchymosis, swelling, and point tenderness at the fracture site are typically seen on examination. A standard foot film series should be obtained.

Management: patient should be placed non–weight bearing for 3 to 5 days in a posterior splint or CAM boot. Indications for orthopedic referrals include open fractures, intraarticular fractures, or multiple metatarsal fractures. First metatarsal fractures with displacement or angulation should also be referred. Second through fifth metatarsal fractures can be managed by a primary care provider as long as there is less than 3 mm displacement and less than 10° angulation in the dorsoplantar plane. Definitive treatment options include SLWC or CAM boot for 6 weeks with progressive weight bearing as tolerated. Repeat imaging should occur at 1 week and at 4 to 6 weeks.[7] After fracture healing, athletes may slowly increase their activity level as pain allows.[5]

Proximal Fifth Metatarsal

Proximal fifth metatarsal fractures are important to recognize and classify correctly, as there is a high complication rate if not managed appropriately.

The proximal fifth metatarsal is divided into 3 regions/zones.

Zone 1: the most proximal region—metatarsal styloid.

Zone 2: the middle region—the metaphyseal-diaphyseal junction includes the joint between the base of the fifth and fourth metatarsals.

Zone 3: the third region—proximal diaphysis.

Patients will have focal tenderness and often will have difficulty bearing weight. zone 1 injuries often occur after an ankle inversion injury. Patients with a zone 3 injury will often describe previous pain in the region. A standard 3-view foot plain film radiograph series should be obtained.

Zone 1/avulsion fractures: treatment options include weight bearing as tolerated in a postop (hard-soled) shoe or low tide CAM boot. Patients only need to limit activities based on symptom control; otherwise, pain can be a guide for return to activity. Refer to orthopedist for greater than 3 mm of displacement, step-off greater than 2 mm on the cuboid articular surface, or if the fracture includes more than 60% of the metatarsal-cuboid joint surface.[7] Physical therapy to address the associated lateral ankle injury is often needed after fracture healing.

Zone 2/Jones fracture management: because of poor blood flow, these injuries often require upwards of 3 to 4 months to heal with conservative management. In addition, there is a high rate of nonunion in nonoperative treatment of Jones fractures, upward of 70%.[36] Given these factors, referral to orthopedics should occur.

Zone 3/stress fractures: these high-risk injuries should always be referred to orthopedics.

TOE FRACTURES

The most common mechanism of injury for toe fracture is axial loading or a crush injury.[5] Patients present with pain, ecchymosis, swelling, and difficulty ambulating.

Management depends on which phalanx is injured. For great toe injuries, referral for surgical evaluation should occur for displaced intraarticular fractures, nondisplaced intraarticular fractures that involve greater than a quarter of the joint space, and all physeal fractures in pediatric patients.[5,7] Conservative management begins with a CAM walking boot for 2 to 3 weeks. After 2 to 3 weeks in the boot, the patient can be transitioned to buddy taping with the use of a rigid-sole shoe for an additional 3 to 4 weeks.[7] Return to sport may take several more weeks.

In lesser toe fractures, nondisplaced fractures can be managed with buddy taping, wearing a rigid sole shoe, and ambulation as tolerated. Patients should follow-up in 1 to 2 weeks to ensure maintained alignment. Buddy taping for 3 to 6 weeks is often required.[5,7] For displaced fractures, reduction should be attempted and managed as discussed earlier. Referral to orthopedics is indicated for open fractures, displaced intraarticular fractures, intraarticular fractures involving more than a quarter of the joint, angulation greater than 10° (mediolateral plane), angulation greater than 20° (dorsoplantar plane), rotational deformity greater than 20°, intraarticular fractures involving more than a quarter of the joint, and physeal fractures.[5,7]

SUMMARY

Appropriate determination of definitive fracture management, either nonoperative or operative, and immobilization is imperative to injury healing. Short-term immobilization of the shoulder and the elbow is often achieved with simple slings or short-term splinting. Gutter splints are often used for phalanx or metacarpal fractures. Carpal bone and distal radius fractures usually require short-term volar splinting with definitive treatment following with a short arm cast. Posterior splints are appropriate for the acute treatment of metatarsal shaft fractures, Jones fractures, and nondisplaced malleolar fracture. CAM walker boots are used for second to fifth metatarsal shaft fractures, zone 1 fractures of the proximal fifth metatarsal fractures, great toe fractures, and nonoperative ankle fractures. Nondisplaced or minimally displaced lesser toe fractures may be managed with buddy taping and a hard-soled shoe.

CLINICS CARE POINTS

- A minimum of 2 views, an AP and lateral, are required to properly assess fracture positioning.
- After a fracture it is critical to evaluate for neurovascular injuries.
- Initial fracture stabilization usually occurs using a splint with casting occurring in 5 to 7 days after initial swelling has improved. After initial stabilization, complicated fractures should be referred to a specialist.
- Indication for surgical referral versus nonoperative management is determined by which bone is fractured, the type of fracture, position of the fracture (angulation, rotation, or displacement) and stability.
- Suspected scaphoid fractures with abnormal radiographs should be immobilized in thumb spica splints and radiographs repeated in 7 to 10 days.
- Stable metacarpal fractures with acceptable angulation should be managed with an ulnar (fourth or fifth metacarpal) or radial (second or third metacarpal) gutter splint for 4 weeks.

DISCLOSURE

The authors have nothing to disclose.

SUPPLEMENTARY DATA

Supplementary data related to this article can be found online at 10.1016/j.pop.2021. 10.007.

REFERENCES

1. Skinner E, Conboy V. Management of common upper limb fractures in adults. Surgery (Oxford) 2019;37(5):258–64.
2. Monica J, Vredenburgh Z, Korsh J, et al. Acute shoulder injuries in adults. Am Fam Physician 2016;94(2):119–27.

3. Kodde IF, Kaas L, Flipsen M, et al. Current concepts in the management of radial head fractures. World J Orthop 2015;6(11):954–60.

4. Boyd AS, Benjamin HJ, Asplund C. Splints and casts: indications and methods. Am Fam Physician 2009;80(5):491–9.

5. Eiff ME, Hatch RL. Fracture management for primary care. 3rd edition. Philadelphia: Elsevier; 2017.

6. Hatch RL, Alsobrook JA, Clugston JR. Diagnosis and management of metatarsal fractures. Am Fam Physician 2007;76:817–26.

7. Bica D, Sprouse RA, Armen J. Diagnosis and management of common foot fractures. Am Fam Physician 2016;93(3):183–91.

8. Ropars M, Thomazeau H, Huten D. Clavicle fractures. Orthopaedics Traumatol Surg Res 2017;103:S53–7.

9. Kancherla VK, Singh A, Anakwenze OA. Management of acute proximal humeral fractures. J Am Acad Orthop Surg 2017;25:42–52.

10. Schumaier A, Grawe B. Proximal humerus fracture: evaluation and management in the elderly patient. Geriatr Orthop Surg Rehabil 2018;9:1–11.

11. Court-Brown CM, Caesar B. Epidemiology of adult fractures: a review. Injury 2006;37(8):691–7.

12. Updegrove GF, Mourad W, Abboud JA. Humeral shaft fractures. J Shoulder Elbow Surg 2018;27:e87–97.

13. Wiegand L, Bernstein J, Ahn J. Fractures in brief: olecranon fractures. Clin Orthop Relat Res 2012;470(12):3637–41.

14. Cai XZ, Yan SG, Giddins G. A systematic review of non-operative treatment of nightstick fractures of the ulna. Bone Joint J 2013;95B(7):952–9.

15. Pulos N, Kakar S. Hand and wrist injuries: common problems and solutions. Clin Sports Med 2018;37:217–43.

16. Ten Berg PW, Drijkoningen T, Strackee SD, et al. Classifications of acute scaphoid fractures; a systematic literature review. J Wrist Surg 2016;5(2):152–9.

17. Abraham MK, Scott S. The emergent evaluation and treatment of hand and wrist injuries. Emerg Med Clin North Am 2010;28(4):789–809.

18. Clementson M, Bjorkman A, Thomsen NO. Acute scaphoid fractures: guidelines for diagnosis and treatment. EFFORT Open Rev 2020;5:96–103.

19. Ko JH, Pet MA, Khouri JS, et al. Management of scaphoid fractures. Plast Reconstr Surg 2017;140(2):333e–46e.

20. Kollitz KM, Hammert WC, Vedder NB, et al. Metacarpal fractures: treatment and complications. Hand (NY) 2014;9(1):16–23.

21. Hung C-Y, Varacallo M, Chang CV. In: StatPearls, editor. Gamekeepers thumb. 2020. Available at: https://www.ncbi.nlm.nih.gov/books/NBK499971/. Accessed January 30, 2021.

22. Borchers JR, Best TM. Common finger fractures and dislocations. Am Fam Physician 2012;85(8):805–10.

23. Elfar J, Mann T. Fracture-dislocations of the proximal interphalangeal joint. J Am Acad Orthop Surg 2013;21(2):88–98.

24. Sprous RA, McLaughling AM, Harris GD. Braces and splints for common musculoskeletal conditions. Am Fam Physician 2018;98(10):570–6.

25. Sikka RS, Dhami R, Dunlay R, et al. Isolated fibular collateral ligament injuries in athletes sports. Med Arthrosc Rev 2015;23(1):17–21.

26. Melvin JS, Mehta S. Patellar fractures in adults. J Am Acad Orthop Surg 2011;19:198–207.

27. Alqarnia N, Goldman RD. Management of toddler's fracture. Can Fam Physician 2018;64:740–1.

28. Adamich JS. Camp, MW. Do toddler's fractures of the tibia require evaluation and management by an orthopedics surgeon routinely? Eur J Emerg Med 2018;25: 423–8.
29. Cepela DJ, Tartaglione JP, Dooley TP, et al. Classifications in brief: salter-harris classification of pediatric physeal fractures. Clin Orthop Relat Res 2016;474: 2531–7.
30. Thomas RA, Henrikus WL. Treatment and outcomes of distal tibia salter harris II fractures. Injury 2020;51:636–41.
31. Stiell IG, Greenberg GH, McKnight RD, et al. Decision rules for the use of radiography in acute ankle injuries. Refinement and prospective validation. JAMA 1993; 269(9):1127–32.
32. Beckenkamp PR, Lin C-WC, Macaskill P, et al. Diagnostic accuracy of the Ottawa Ankle and Midfoot Rules: a systematic review with meta-analysis. Br J Sports Med 2017;51(6):504–10.
33. Egol KA, Koval KJ, Zuckerman JD. Handbook of fractures. 6th edition. Philadelphia: Wolters Kluwer Health; 2019.
34. Nickless JT, Alland JA. High ankle sprains: easy to miss, so follow these tips. The J Fam Pract 2019;68(3):E5–13.
35. Hunt KJ, Phisitukul P, Pirolo J, et al. High ankle sprains and syndesmotic injuries in athletes. J Am Acad Orthop Surg 2015;23(11):661–73.
36. Ruta DJ, Jones PD. Fracture management in athletes. Orthop Clin N Am 2020;51: 541–53.

Point-of-Care Ultrasound for Musculoskeletal Injection and Clinical Evaluation

Jared Dubey, DO[a],*, Brian Shian, MD[b]

KEYWORDS

- Point-of-care ultrasound • Primary care ultrasound • Ultrasound-guided injection
- Abdominal aortic aneurysm screening • Deep vein thrombosis evaluation
- Basic echocardiography • Cellulitis • Abscess

KEY POINTS

- Technological advances have brought portable and affordable ultrasound to the bedside, with primary care poised to become the next field of medicine to adopt POCUS widely.
- POCUS improves patient satisfaction, lowers cost of care, hastens diagnosis, and expedites treatment.
- POCUS may be used for a variety of diagnostic and procedural purposes including musculoskeletal-guided injection and evaluation of the heart, lungs, vasculature, skin, and soft tissue.

 Video content accompanies this article at http://www.primarycare.theclinics.com.

INTRODUCTION

Poised between an extension of the physical examination and a limited diagnostic study, Point-of-Care Ultrasound (POCUS) has transformed what is possible, diagnostically and therapeutically, at the bedside. Studies have concluded that POCUS improves patient satisfaction, lowers the cost of care, lessens the use of ionizing radiation, and reduces the time to definitive treatment.[1–4] With these dramatic benefits in mind, POCUS has already been widely adopted by Emergency Medicine and Critical Care. With each technological advancement that ultrasound makes, the breadth of clinical adoption grows. Handheld devices are now bringing bedside ultrasound to the primary care clinic setting (**Table 1**).

[a] Department of Family Medicine and Community Health, University of Wisconsin School of Medicine and Public Health, 3209 Dryden Drive, Madison, WI 53704, USA; [b] Department of Family Medicine, University of Iowa Carver College of Medicine, Pomerantz Family Pavilion, 200 Hawkins Drive, Iowa City, IA 52242, USA
* Corresponding author.
E-mail address: jdubey@wisc.edu

Prim Care Clin Office Pract 49 (2022) 163–189
https://doi.org/10.1016/j.pop.2021.10.011
0095-4543/22/© 2021 Elsevier Inc. All rights reserved.
primarycare.theclinics.com

Table 1	
Example POCUS applications in primary care	
AAA Screening	Is There An Aneurysm?
Cardiac	Is there LV systolic dysfunction?
Soft Tissue	Is there an abscess or foreign body?
MSK	Is there a tendon rupture?
Procedures	Is the needle in the joint/avoiding vessels?
RUQ	Are there gallstones?
Pulmonary	Is there pulmonary edema?
Renal	Is there hydronephrosis?
Vascular	Is there a DVT?
Obstetric	Is there an IUP? Gestational age?

Abbreviations: DVT, deep vein thrombosis; IUP, intrauterine pregnancy; LV, left ventricular; MSK, musculoskeletal; RUQ, right upper quadrant.

Limitations

While expediency gives POCUS an advantage over sonographer performed and radiologist interpreted ultrasound, POCUS is not a replacement for such scans, which unlike POCUS are comprehensive and protocoled. When POCUS is not able to answer the clinical query or incidental findings are appreciated, referral for comprehensive imaging or consultation is advised. This article is intended to serve as a reference and review to augment hands-on training in the use of POCUS.

Equipment

Both hand-held and portable cart-based machines can be used for POCUS. Handheld devices offer the advantages of being extremely portable and easy to clean, whereas cart-based machines typically offer superior image quality and more advanced image processing capability.

The following are the 4 main transducer types: curvilinear, linear, phased array, and endocavitary. Each varies slightly in footprint and in how ultrasound beams are transmitted.

- Curvilinear probes emit low-frequency waves from a curved rectangular footprint in a diverging path. These transducers are best suited for imaging structures beyond 5 cm depth.
- Linear probes generate high-frequency waves in straight lines from a flat rectangular footprint and are best suited for imaging more superficial structures (ie, <5 cm) and are the best choice for procedural guidance such as needle visualization.
- Phased array probes generate pulsed, low-frequency waves from a small triangular footprint, which allows for a wide field of view from a small footprint and also allows for more accurate imaging of moving structures, making the phased array transducer ideal for cardiac imaging.
- Intracavitary probes combine high-frequency waves and a small convex footprint, which makes them ideal for transvaginal, transrectal, or intraoral imaging.
- Lastly, there are now microchip-based transducers that use a single probe to emulate the function of all 4 probes described earlier. This can be a significant advantage when it comes to portability and cost. However, the footprint of the probe, which does not change, can make certain applications challenging (**Fig. 1**).

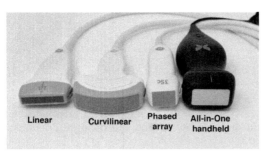

Fig. 1. Transducer types. (*From* pocus101.com; with permission.)

Imaging Modes

- *B-mode* (sometimes called 2-D mode) generates the classic black and white cross images typically associated with ultrasound.
- *M-mode* shows the change over time along a one-dimensional cross-section (single line) of the 2-D image.
- *Color Doppler* overlays color to indicate motion. This is especially useful for showing blood flow through vessels.
- *Spectral Doppler* applies Doppler analysis to a single point or line to generate a waveform that represents motion at that point or along that line over time.

Ultrasound Safety

Ultrasound does not generate any ionizing radiation and is considered extremely safe. Although absorption of ultrasound waves does generate heat, the effect is small. Because of theoretic risk related to this thermal impact, especially on sensitive tissue such as the eye or early embryo, the As Low As Reasonably Achievable (ALARA) principle is considered best practice. Practically speaking, this means avoiding prolonged single-point scanning of the eye and fetus, especially when using Doppler imaging, because of its use of waves with increased power.

Orientation

Successful use of POCUS requires successful image acquisition and accurate interpretation. The first step to image interpretation and acquisition is proper orientation. To begin with, consistent patient, provider, and ultrasound machine positioning should be used. Traditionally, the operator sits or stands to the patient's right side, with her right hand operating the probe, whereas the left hand operates the ultrasound machine, which sits in front of the operator. Once the patient, provider, and machine are properly arranged, screen orientation must be considered. By convention, the top of the screen always corresponds to the probe, with the image toward the top of the screening representing superficial structures with deeper structures seen more toward the bottom of the screen. To orient left versus right of the screen, the provider must be aware of the orientation marker on the probe and the orientation marker on the screen. By convention, for all ultrasounds aside from cardiac, the orientation marker will be found on the left side of the screen (provider's left when facing the screen). Echocardiography by convention uses the opposite orientation (ie, orientation marker on right side of the screen). The orientation marker on the screen aligns with the orientation marker on the probe. Thus, if the probe is held in the sagittal plane, with the marker toward the patient's head, the left side of the screen will show more superior structures and the right side of the screen more inferior (**Fig. 2**).

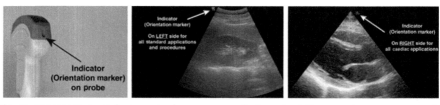

Fig. 2. Orientation marker on probe corresponds to orientation marker on screen. By convention, standard and cardiac imaging use opposite orientations. (*From* pocus101. com; with permission.)

Transducer Movements

The following 4 main transducer motions are described: sliding, rotating, tilting, and rocking. Sliding is the movement of the entire transducer without changing the angle of relationship between the transducer and the patient. Rotating is keeping the center of the transducer stationary, while rotating it along its midline axis. Tilting is also referred to as fanning or sweeping and is performed by maintaining a constant long axis of transducer contact and tilting the transducer back and forth across this axis. Rocking is done by maintaining a constant short axis of the transducer contact and pushing one end of the transducer or the other into the patient to move the ultrasound beam toward or away from structures in plan with the current image (**Fig. 3**).

Artifacts

Artifacts are images that do not correspond to true anatomic structures. Artifacts occur in all imaging modalities. In ultrasound, artifacts often offer valuable information about anatomy, even if they are not directly representative of that anatomy.

Reverberation

Reverberation artifact occurs when an ultrasound beam bounces multiple times between 2 highly reflective surfaces before returning to the probe. This results in the probe receiving the reflected signal at regular time intervals corresponding to the number of reflections that the wave has executed. Because the ultrasound machine assumes all signals received reflect only one time, signals returning later are considered deeper structures. Thus, the reverberation phenomenon produces a series of bright hyperechoic lines at regular depth intervals. This artifact is seen when scanning the lung. In this case, skin and the pleural line form 2 reflective surfaces that the

Cardinal transducer manipulation/movement
(Sliding, Tilting, Rotating, and Rocking)

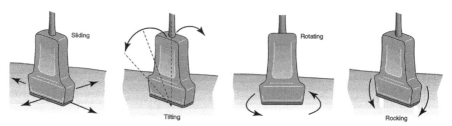

Fig. 3. Transducer movements sliding, tilting, rotating, and rocking. (*From* pocus101.com; with permission.)

ultrasound wave will bounce between a variable number of times before returning to the probe. As we will see in the lung section, this generates the classic A-line pattern, which indicates normal air-filled lung tissue (**Fig. 4**).

Mirror artifact
When a highly reflective surface, such as diaphragm, exists deep into an organ being imaged (eg, the liver), some of the ultrasound waves will bounce off the diaphragm, then bounce off the liver back to the diaphragm, before finally bouncing back to the transducer. Because the machine equates time with depth, an additional liver will be visible deep to the diaphragm (**Fig. 5**).

Edge artifact
Edge artifact occurs because of ultrasound waves being refracted (ie, deflected) as they pass by the edge of smooth curved structures. Because of this deflection, there is an area of absent signal return just deep to the edge, causing a hypoechoic or anechoic streak to appear (**Fig. 6**).

Shadowing
Shadowing occurs because contrary to the assumptions made by the machine, attenuation of sound wave energy varies by tissue type. As waves encounter highly attenuating tissue, energy is lost, leading to a hypoechoic or anechoic region deep to the highly attenuating structure. Rib shadows or the shadow deep to a gallstone are good examples of this (**Fig. 7**).

Posterior enhancement
When waves pass through tissues with very low attenuation, such as water or other fluids, the waves returning from deep to that structure will have more energy than waves returning from adjacent tissues at the same depth that had to pass through a relatively more attenuating tissue. This leads to a brighter/more hyperechoic appearance to structures deep to fluid or cystic structures (**Fig. 8**).

MUSCULOSKELETAL INJECTION
Overview

Musculoskeletal injections, including intra-articular, intrabursal, peritendon, and perineural injections, are frequently performed in the clinical setting for diagnostic and therapeutic purposes.[5] Common injectates include corticosteroid, dextrose, and platelet-rich plasma.

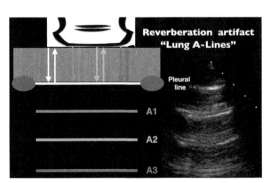

Fig. 4. Reverberation artifact producing so-called A-line pattern in normal lung. (*From* pocus101.com; with permission.)

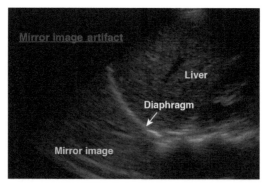

Fig. 5. Mirror artifact produces the illusion of liver tissue above the diaphragm. (*From* pocus101.com; with permission.)

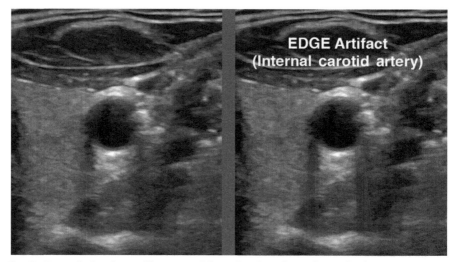

Fig. 6. Hypoechoic edge artifact caused by refraction along the wall of an artery. (*From* pocus101.com; with permission.)

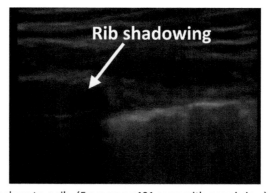

Fig. 7. Shadowing deep to a rib. (*From* pocus101.com; with permission.)

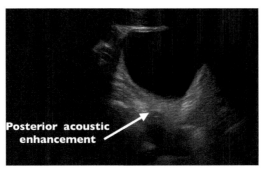

Fig. 8. Posterior enhancement deep to the bladder. (*From* pocus101.com; with permission.)

Traditionally, a palpation-guided approach (PGA) is used. PGA involves inherent risk for inaccurate needle placement and accidental injury to surrounding structures. To avoid such complications, image-guided approaches are gaining popularity, especially with ultrasound guidance due to technological advancement, accessibility, portability, nonionizing radiation, and lower cost.[6] In addition, evidence supports that ultrasound-guided injection (USGI) is less painful and has better outcomes compared with PGA[7]

USGI procedure checklist

1. Obtain informed consent from the patient or his/her durable power of attorney.
2. Gather supplies as listed in **Box 1**.
3. Place the patient in a comfortable position with the target area well exposed and easily accessible.
4. Preform preprocedure ultrasound to identify target, plane of approach, and anatomy to avoid.
5. Mark the probe position and site of needle entry.
6. Clean and disinfect the injection site.
7. Prep the proper amount of injectate.
8. Anesthetize the injection site with ethyl chloride or a small amount (1–3 mL) of rapid-acting local anesthetic using a 27- to 30-gauge needle. (optional)
9. Under direct ultrasound visualization, advance the needle to the target area and inject the solution.

Box 1
USGI supply list

Items
- Gloves
- Gauze
- Alcohol wipe
- Skin prep solution, like Povidone-iodine swab
- Adhesive bandage
- Ethyl chloride spray (optional)
- Medications
- Needles & Syringes
- Test tube or culture material if needed
- Assistant if needed
- Ultrasound machine with sterile cover and gel

10. Withdraw the needle, clean the point of entry, and apply a proper dressing.
11. Give the patient postinjection instructions.
12. Document the procedure in the patient's chart.

As most musculoskeletal structures are not very deep, a regular high-frequency linear (HFL) probe (>10 mHz) or a hockey stick linear probe, if equipped, can be used for USGI. An exception to this is the hip joint, especially in larger patients, for which the curvilinear probe may be needed.

Before the injection, scan the targeted area in transverse and longitudinal to orient to the patient's anatomy. It is generally wise to use the color Doppler mode to ensure no vessels lie in the intended needle pathway.

Needle guidance can be achieved using either an in-plane or out-of-plane approach. When possible, we favor an in-plane approach, advancing the needle in the plane of the ultrasound image, thereby allowing for visualization of the entire needle as it is advanced. In some cases, an in-plane approach is not possible and an out-of-plane approach is needed. Out-of-plane involves the needle traveling perpendicularly to the plane of the ultrasound image. The transducer can be fanned just proximal to the target tissue and the needle advanced until the tip is seen, then the transducer is fanned back to the target and the needle is slowly advanced until the needle tip is visualized at the target.

There are a variety of USGI approaches for a given joint or site. A discussion of all possible approaches is beyond the scope of this article. Thus, for a given site, only one commonly used approach based on literature and the author's experience will be addressed here.

Selected Targets

Acromioclavicular joint

For the anterior in-plane approach to the acromioclavicular joint (ACJ), the patient is placed in the supine position with some supporting material under the upper back to somewhat elevate the shoulder as described in the literature.[8] An HFL probe is placed short axis to the clavicle and moved laterally until the bony acoustic landmarks of the clavicle disappear and the AC joint comes into view. Then a small-gauged needle is introduced in an in-plane anterior-to-posterior fashion under direct real-time guidance to anesthetize the skin and enter the ACJ, the syringe is exchanged, and the medication is delivered under USG (**Fig. 9**).

Subacromial subdeltoid bursa (SASDB)

For USGI, the lateral approach is commonly used.[8]

The patient is placed in a decubitus position and lies on the unaffected side. Under sterile fashion, an HFL probe is placed adjacent to the lateral part of the acromion process, along the long axis of supraspinatus tendon in the anatomic coronal plane. Once the subacromial subdeltoid bursa (SASDB) is identified, a needle can be introduced under ultrasound guidance to the SASDB, which is between the deltoid muscle and the supraspinatus tendon. A small amount of local anesthetic can be injected to confirm the needle placement inside the SASDB because injection inside the SASDB causes hydrodissection. Once the placement is confirmed, exchange syringes to deliver the right amount of steroid with or without additional local anesthetics (**Fig. 10**).

Glenohumeral joint

The posterior approach is frequently used in USGI for the glenohumeral joint, which can be best visualized using an HFL or a curvilinear-array probe placed short axis to the joint in the oblique axial plane. The patient is generally laying in the decubitus

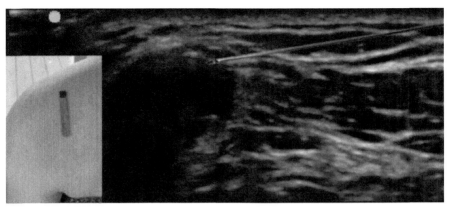

Fig. 9. Acromioclavicular joint ultrasound-guided injection—anterior approach.

position on the contralateral side, slightly leaning forward and the affected should somewhat adducted. Under sterile fashion, the proper acoustic window is obtained to identify the humeral head, the edge of the glenoid fossa, and labium. It is important to note that because of the hyaline cartilage from the humeral head, a thin black anechoic layer may exist between the muscle and the humeral bony cortex. Once the structures are identified, a properly sized needle is introduced via an in-plane anterolateral-to-posteromedial approach to reach the area above the hyaline cartilage that is lateral to the labrum to avoid puncturing the labrum. Once the needle placement is confirmed, the desired amount of medication mixture can be injected. In the case of adhesive capsulitis, higher volumes of injectate may be desired to produce capsular distension. Volumes of up to 20 mL have been reported without capsule rupture and with good clinical outcomes[8] (**Fig. 11**).

Long head of the biceps brachii tendon

The long head of the biceps brachii tendon (LHBBT) can be easily identified in the intertubercular groove under ultrasound evaluation.

The injection target is the space between the tendon and its sheath, not the tendon itself. The anterior in-plane method on the short axis of the LHBBT is generally used.[8] The patient is predominantly placed in the supine position with the arm in mild external rotation. Under sterile fashion, a color doppler evaluation might be needed to locate

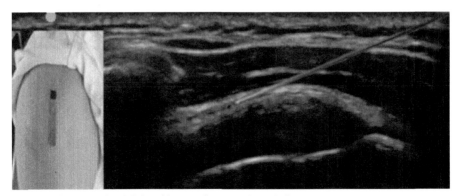

Fig. 10. Subacromial subdeltoid bursa ultrasound-guided injection.

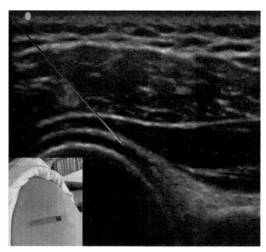

Fig. 11. Glenohumeral joint ultrasound-guided joint injection.

any close by vascular structure, then with 2D mode, the LHBBT is identified, and a properly sized needle is introduced under real-time guidance to reach the space between the LHBBT and its sheath. Once the placement is confirmed, the desired amount of injectate can be pushed in (**Fig. 12**).

De Quervain tenosynovitis
De Quervain syndrome can involve the abductor pollicis longus and/or extensor pollicis brevis tendons, which are located just palmar to the radial styloid. The superficial radial nerve travels from palmar to dorsal just proximal to the radial styloid and should be identified before injection.

The patient can be seated with the forearm supported and the ulnar side of the wrist resting on a rolled-up towel to create ulnar deviation. An HFL probe is then placed at

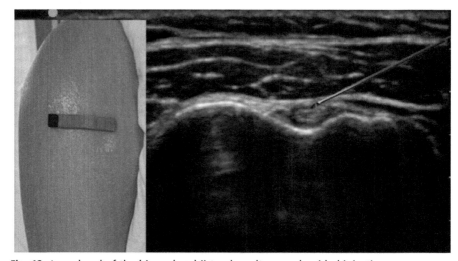

Fig. 12. Long head of the biceps brachii tendon ultrasound-guided injection.

the radial styloid process, perpendicular to the tendons. Color Doppler may be used to identify vasculature. A properly sized needle is then introduced from the dorsal side. Once the needle reaches the space between the tendons and their sheath, the desired amount of injectate can be delivered[9,10] (**Fig. 13**).

Carpal tunnel syndrome

The in-plane ulnar approach is frequently used for carpal tunnel syndrome injection in which the injectate is delivered above and below the median nerve under ultrasound guidance to avoid accidental nerve injury. The patient is seated or in the supine position with the forearm supinated and the wrist rested on a rolled-up towel to create wrist extension. Under sterile fashion, an HFL probe is placed across the wrist crease. Next, identify the median nerve and flexor tendons. A small gauge needle is then passed from the ulnar aspect of the carpal tunnel to a position anterior to the median nerve. Following that, injection of solution peels the nerve from the overlying flexor retinaculum via hydrodissection. Then, the needle is retracted and reintroduced to a position posterior to the median nerve. The injectates delivered will separate the deep surface of the median nerve from the more deeply positioned hyperechoic flexor tendons[9] (**Figs. 14 and 15**).

Hip joint

The hip joint is a relatively deep structure and a curved linear array probe is frequently needed. The patient is placed in a supine position with the affected hip laterally rotated and the ipsilateral knee slightly flexed. Under sterile fashion, the probe is generally placed in the long-axis plane of the femoral neck, starting from the midpoint of the inguinal ligament, then sliding distally. Once the femoral head and neck are well visualized on the screen, scanning slightly to the medial side to notice the location of the major vessels and nerve to assess the safety of the needle entering the pathway. Color Doppler mode may be helpful. Once the vessels and nerves are identified, go back to visualize the femoral head and neck again; the junction at the neck and head under the joint capsule is the targeted location for injection. Using an in-plane mode, a properly sized needle is introduced to reach the position. Once the placement is confirmed, the desired amount of injectate is delivered[11] (**Fig. 16**).

Great trochanteric bursa

The author likes to use the dynamic USGI trochanteric bursal injection.[12] The patient is placed in a decubitus position on the unaffected side. A HFL probe or a curved linear

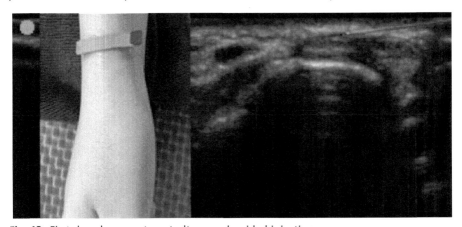

Fig. 13. First dorsal compartment ultrasound-guided injection.

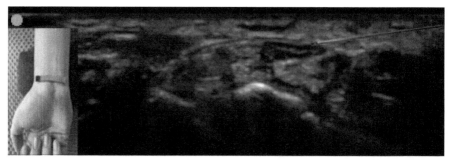

Fig. 14. Carpal tunnel syndrome ultrasound-guided injection.

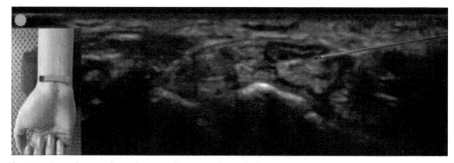

Fig. 15. Carpal tunnel syndrome ultrasound-guided injection.

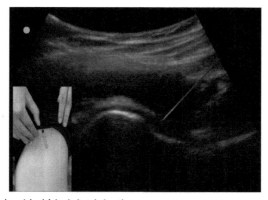

Fig. 16. Ultrasound-guided hip joint injection.

probe can be placed transversely to locate the lateral trochanteric surface just distal to the tip of the greater trochanter. The patient should be instructed to externally rotate the ipsilateral hip; this will help to locate the trochanteric bursa space between the gluteus medius and the fascia lata/iliotibial tract. Using an in-plane posterior approach, an appropriate needle is advanced through the iliotibial band (or adjacent fascia lata) and into the trochanteric bursa space to deliver the injectate (**Fig. 17**).

Knee joint
The suprapatellar approach is described. The patient is supine with the affected knee slightly bent, resting on a rolled-up towel or other supporting material. A HFL probe is placed transversely just above the superior edge of the patella. The suprapatellar recess can be visualized, especially if any effusion is present. Once the target is identified, using an in-plane mode, a needle can be inserted and guided to the recess, the injectate should be injected with no resistance and flow distally into the patellofemoral joint[13] (**Fig. 18**).

First metatarsophalangeal joint
The first metatarsophalangeal (MTP) joint is superficial and small. The patient lies supine with the affected foot flat on the table. The clinician then positions himself or herself at the caudal side of the table, facing the patient, with the ultrasound machine adjacent to the examining table.[14] Under sterile fashion, an HFL probe is placed longitudinally over the dorsal aspect of the MTP joint to identify the extensor hallucis longus tendon, then moved medially or laterally, so that no overlying structures impedes access to the joint capsule. Using an in-plane approach, a properly sized needle should pass through the superficial structures then enter the joint capsule to deliver the injectate (**Fig. 19**).

CARDIAC
Overview

There is perhaps no application better suited to ultrasound than evaluation of the heart. Indeed, echocardiography has been an essential tool in the field of cardiology for decades.[15] Studies have shown that with limited training, physicians can identify

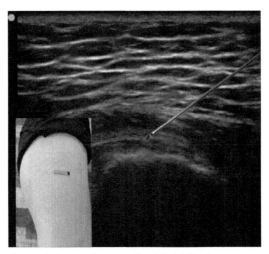

Fig. 17. Greater trochanteric bursa ultrasound-guided injection.

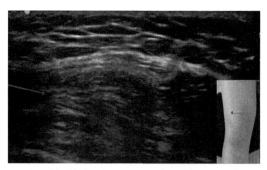

Fig. 18. Knee ultrasound-guided injection—superolateral approach.

left ventricular (LV) systolic dysfunction, LV enlargement, LV hypertrophy, right ventricular enlargement, left atrial enlargement (LAE), severe valve dysfunction, IVC dilatation, and pericardial effusions.[16–19] These pathologic changes to cardiac structure and/or function can be identified with ultrasound before symptoms or physical examination findings manifest.[20] Furthermore, in the case of many commonly seen acute complaints, which generate broad differential diagnoses (such as dyspnea or cough), POCUS can rule in or rule out not to miss diagnoses, such as decompensated heart failure and is especially valuable in conjunction with lung ultrasound findings.[1,20,21]

Limitations and Challenges

Device capability, operator skill, and patient factors have the potential to limit the use of cardiac POCUS. In some cases, patient factors (such as habitus or chronic obstructive pulmonary disease) and/or operator skills prevent the acquisition of quality images. In other cases, such as assessment of valvular function or filling pressures (which are routinely included in comprehensive echocardiography), technological limitations and/or operator skills may prevent adequate assessment. When bedside POCUS fails or results are ambiguous, referral for comprehensive imaging or specialist consultation is advised (**Fig. 20**).

Selected Assessments

Assessment of left ventricular ejection fraction using E-point septal separation
Myocardial thickening, endocardial excursion, and E-point septal separation (EPSS) are all parameters that may be considered when assessing LV function using POCUS. For the purposes of this text, we focus on the EPSS method, which requires only one

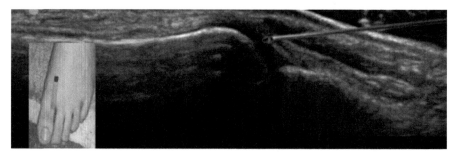

Fig. 19. First metatarsophalangeal ultrasound-guided joint.

View	Description	Picture	US image
Parasternal long	3rd or 4th intercostal (IC) space, indicator pointed towards patient's right shoulder[a]	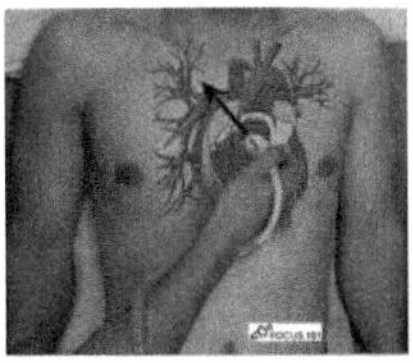	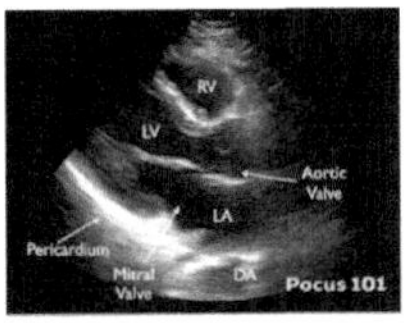
Parasternal short	3rd or 4th IC space, indicator pointed toward patient's right shoulder[a]	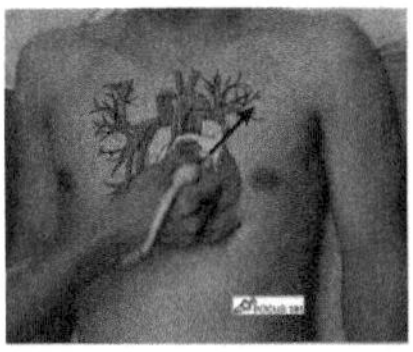	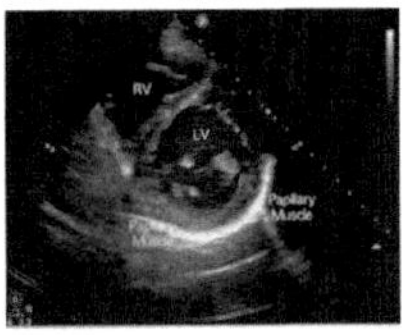
Apical 4 chamber	PMI, indicator towards patient's left side[a]	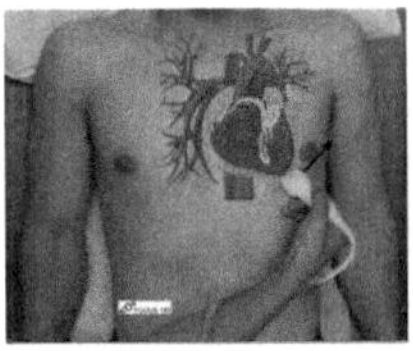	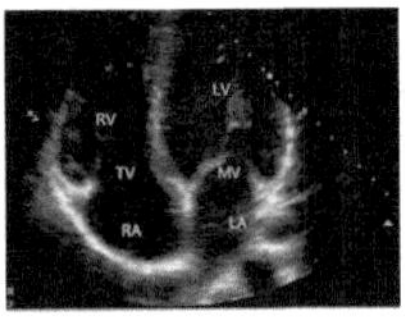
Subcostal	Subxyphoid, indicator pointed towards patient's left side[a]	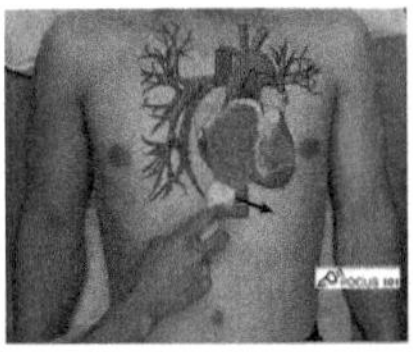	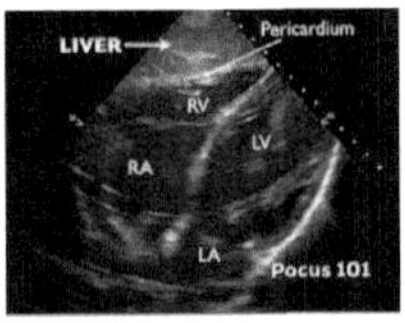
IVC	Subxyphoid, indicator pointed towards patient's head[a]	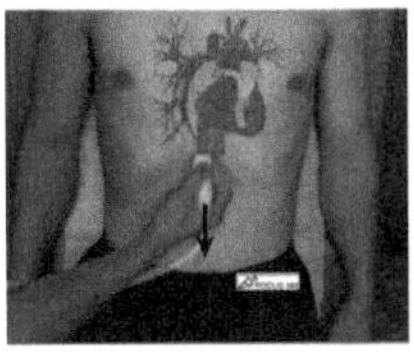	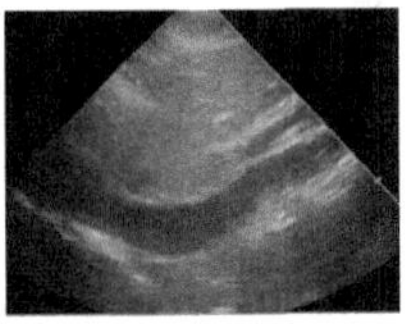

[a]when in cardiac mode. If in another mode, rotate the probe 180 degrees.

Fig. 20. Cardiac POCUS views table. (*Figures from* pocus101.com; with permission.)

view and has a sensitivity and specificity estimated to be 69% to 94% and 88% to 94%, respectively.[20]

EPSS refers to the minimal distance between the tip of the anterior leaflet of the mitral valve (E-point) and the interventricular septum during the cardiac cycle and is assessed in the parasternal long-axis view in diastole. An EPSS $\leq$ 1 cm is normal and is consistent with an LVEF greater than 40%. Conversely, an EPSS >1 cm suggests an LV systolic dysfunction with an EF $\leq$ 40%. When available, M-mode may help with this visualization (Videos 1 and 2).

Assessment of LAE
LAE occurs as a consequence of sustained or episodically elevated left atrial (LA) pressures, is an important marker for cardiac disease, and is an independent risk factor for all-cause mortality.[21,22] Although the most accurate methods for measuring LA size involve sophisticated and precise echocardiographic analysis, POCUS providers can effectively rule in or rule out moderate-severe LAE with a qualitative assessment of the left atrium-to-aorta diastolic diameter ratio.[20,21,23] At the end of diastole, using either visual estimation or m-mode, the diameters of the left atrium and the aorta at the sinuses of Valsalva are compared. A ratio greater than 1 suggests moderate or severe LAE. This method has been shown to have a sensitivity and specificity of 75% and 72%, respectively, when compared to standard echo.[23] Caveats to this approach include asymmetric LA enlargement (ie, with maintained anteroposterior diameter) and aortic root dilation, both of which may lead to false negatives.

LOWER EXTREMITY DEEP VEIN THROMBOSIS
Overview

Abundant literature has investigated the use of POCUS for deep vein thrombosis (DVT) diagnosis. Multiple studies and meta-analyses have demonstrated sensitivities and specificities above 90% when compared to technologist performed and radiologist interpreted ultrasound.[24,25]

Most DVTs involve the common femoral vein (CFV) or popliteal vein (PV), but isolated thrombosis in the femoral vein (FV), deep femoral vein (DFV), or distal leg can occur. Fortunately, distal DVTs are unlikely to embolize and may not need to be treated. For those whose clots will grow and present embolic risk, the literature supports a strategy of rescanning higher risk patients in 1 week.[26]

2-Point compression
Consistent with the fact that most of the clinically relevant DVTs involve the CFV or PV, recent studies support a simplified 2-point compression (2PC) approach that involves imaging the CFV and PVs only. Whereas, the traditional strategy includes the FV as well and is known as 3-point compression (3PC). A 2019 meta-analysis[25] of 17 studies concluded that both 2PC and 3PC have sensitivity and specificity of over 90%, with similar false-negative rates of ~4%.

Integrated decision making
As with any other test, ultrasound results must be interpreted in context with consideration given to pretest probability based on history and examination. In addition, d-dimer assessment may be used to further risk stratify.

One popular algorithm, which was validated by a multicenter prospective trial[27] of over 1000 patients, incorporates pretest probability (Well's score), D-dimer, and 2PC or comprehensive US for low-risk and high-risk patients, respectively. Unfortunately, D-dimer is often not available as a rapid test at the point of care, and obtaining same-day comprehensive ultrasound imparts logistical challenges and increased cost on the patient and the health care system.

Therefore, the author favors the approach described by Borneman and colleagues.[28] In this approach, patients with low pretest probability and negative 2PC are ruled out. When 2PC is negative but there is moderate or high pretest probability, d-dimer is measured. If d-dimer is negative, DVT is ruled out. If d-dimer is positive, 2PC is repeated in 1 week. A prospective cohort study of 1700 patients[26] supports the fact that this strategy will effectively catch progression of isolated distal or femoral vein thrombosis into the popliteal or CFVs, respectively (**Fig. 21**).

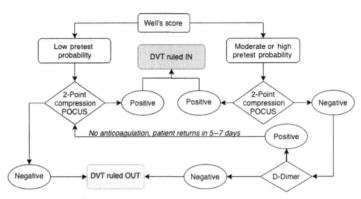

Fig. 21. DVT evaluation algorithm.

Performing the 2PC ultrasound
The patient should be supine with the entire lower extremity exposed, with slight hip abduction, hip external rotation, and knee flexion (frog leg position). Using a HFL probe, scan the CFV from the saphenous confluence until it splits into the DFV and FV, applying compression every 1 to 2 cm. Compression is applied with the probe directly, just enough to start to see the artery change shape. The study is positive if the walls of the vein do not completely collapse and "kiss" each other or if a thrombus is directly visualized. Next, scan and compress the PV, being sure to visualize from the mid popliteal fossa (where the PV is superficial to the popliteal artery) until the trifurcation into the leg veins (Videos 3–6).

ABDOMINAL AORTIC ANEURYSM SCREENING

One-time Abdominal aortic aneurysm (AAA) screening is recommended for men aged 65 to 75 years who have ever smoked and is associated with a 35% reduction in AAA-related mortality.[29] However, it is estimated that only 15% of eligible patients complete this potentially lifesaving imaging.[30] Fortunately, literature supports the fact that AAA screening with POCUS has excellent diagnostic performance compared with comprehensive ultrasound. A meta-analysis of 7 studies, which included a total of 655 patients, determined a sensitivity and specificity of 99% and 98%, respectively.[31]

The proximal, mid, and distal portions of the aorta should be visualized in transverse and longitudinal views. Measurement is made in transverse view from outer wall to outer wall. A normal abdominal aorta is ≤ 3 cm in diameter. Bowel gas is the most common challenge to obtaining images. When gas obscures adequate visualization, persistent pressure is applied and bowel often moves out of the way. Having patients fast for 8 to 10 hours before the scan is another useful strategy to improve chances of success (**Fig. 22**).

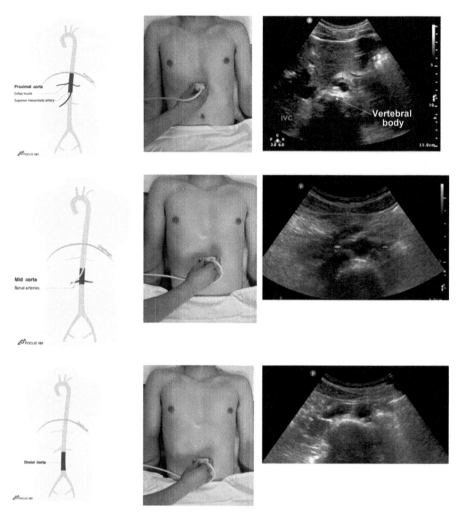

Fig. 22. Proximal, mid, and distal aorta scanning positions with normal findings. (*Adapted from* pocus101.com; with permission.)

PULMONARY

Although it may seem counterintuitive to use ultrasound to image the lung, given the high attenuation properties of air, pulmonary POCUS is an extremely useful tool that outperforms chest x-ray for a number of important diagnostic findings, such as pleural effusion, pneumothorax, pneumonia, and pulmonary edema.[32–34]

Normal lung ultrasound has 2 defining features: lung sliding and an A-line pattern. Lung sliding is the movement between the parietal and visceral pleura. If lung sliding is not seen, it indicates either air between the 2 layers of pleura (ie, a pneumothorax) or adhesion between the layers of pleura (as can be seen with fibrosis or inflammation). An A-line pattern is a reverberation artifact that is produced by the reflection of ultrasound waves back and forth between the skin-transducer interface and the pleura. Thus, in a normal lung, there is no information coming back to the transducer from the lung parenchyma at all (Video 7).

When the septa between alveoli become edematous (due to increased hydrostatic pressure or inflammation), ultrasound waves penetrate the parenchyma and a B-line pattern is seen. B-lines are another type of artifact related to reverberation that occurs when waves bounce around within fluid before returning to the transducer. When a pleural effusion is present, ultrasound waves are transmitted through the effusion and anechoic (black) structure is seen, sometimes with a consolidated lung deep to the effusion, which appears like a solid organ and can represent pneumonia with a parapneumonic effusion or a pleural effusion with lung atelectasis (Video 8; **Fig. 23**).

SOFT-TISSUE INFECTION
Overview

POCUS has been shown to improve diagnostic accuracy and leads to improved management decisions in patients with soft-tissue infection (STIs), especially in cases of indeterminate clinical assessment.[35,36] A HFL probe is typically used. Familiarity with shadowing, posterior enhancement, dirty shadowing due to air, and reverberation artifact are essential for accurate interpretation.

In healthy tissue, skin appears as a thin echogenic layer, whereas subcutaneous fatty tissue is generally hypoechoic with randomly distributed hyperechoic fibrous septa between the fat globules. The fascial planes are hyperechoic and muscle has a characteristic striated appearance. Vascular structures appear anechoic. Nerves appear as hypoechoic fascicles embedded in hyperechoic connective tissue[37] (**Fig. 24**).

Cellulitis

The sonographic findings of cellulitis vary depending on the location and severity. They may start with thickening and increased echogenicity of the involved layers of soft tissue, especially the skin and subcutaneous layers. This progresses to hypoechoic strands in between the hyperechoic fat lobules due to edema and fluid collection between tissues, forming what is known as "cobblestoning"[37,38] (see **Fig. 20**). Importantly, cobblestoning itself does not necessarily mean cellulitis, but rather the presence of soft tissue edema, which may be the result of alternative etiologies, such as gout, superficial thrombophlebitis, congestive heart failure, cirrhosis, nephrotic syndrome, venous insufficiency, or lymphedema. Color or power Doppler imaging may help identify hyperemia within the subcutaneous tissues, suggesting an inflammatory component, which is usually not a feature of noninfectious forms of edema.[37]

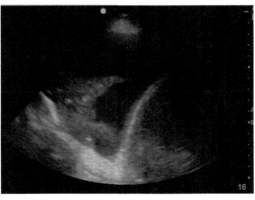

Fig. 23. Pleural effusion with collapsed lung tissue. (*From* pocus101.com; with permission.)

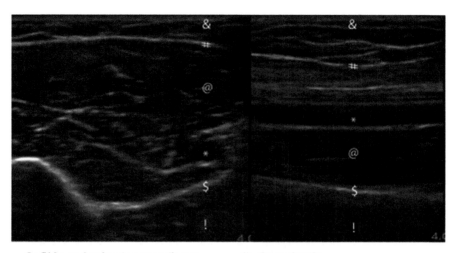

&: Skin and subcutaneous tissue   #: Deep fascia
@: Muscle $: Bony cortex
*: Blood vessel   !: Postacoustic shadow

Fig. 24. Normal soft tissue layers on ultrasound.

However, a detailed history and thorough physical examination are keys to differentiating these conditions from each other (**Fig. 25**).

Abscesses

POCUS of STI is particularly helpful in identifying abscesses. In cases where physical examination is equivocal, POCUS distinguishes abscess from cellulitis and leads to a change in management in 10% to 25% of cases.[39,40] Owing to tissue destruction and fluid (pus) collection, sizable abscesses have distinct sonographic findings on POCUS. They are commonly located in the subcutaneous layer in somewhat spherical shape with irregular borders (see **Fig. 5**). The margins can be highly variable—some may be well circumscribed, and the others may be difficult to discern because of partial blending with surrounding tissues. The interior appearance of an abscess is also highly variable depending on its location, maturity, and whether the necrotic tissue is liquefied. For a mature abscess with liquefied necrotic tissue and pus, an anechoic or hypoechoic complex fluid collection with or without loculations is the classic finding

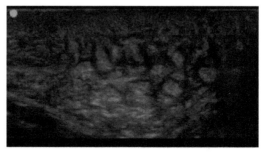

Fig. 25. Cobblestoning in cellulitis.

and is easy to differentiate from the surrounding tissues. Not uncommonly, especially in the early stages, an abscess on ultrasound can be hyperechoic or isoechoic, which may be mistaken as cellulitis by a less experienced provider. A variable number of internal echoes from necrotic debris are seen. Other sonographic findings of abscesses include hyperechoic sediment, septa, loculations, posterior acoustic enhancement, and hyperechoic adjacent subcutaneous tissue. Gentle compression of the abscess with the transducer may show movement or "swirling" of purulent material. Power or color Doppler sonography usually shows hyperemia in the walls of abscesses and immediate surrounding tissues[37,41] (**Fig. 26**).

Other STI Complications

POCUS can detect air in soft tissue and act as a screening test in patients at high risk for subcutaneous air from conditions such as necrotizing fasciitis and gas gangrene.[42] Sonographic findings suggestive of necrotizing fasciitis include marked thickening of the subcutaneous tissues, distorted and thickened fascial layers, and an anechoic fluid collection measuring greater than 4 mm along the deep fascia. In addition, the detection of gas, visualized as acoustic shadowing or reverberation artifacts within the subcutaneous tissues, is pathognomonic for necrotizing fasciitis (see **Fig. 4**). Unlike cellulitis, the inflammatory changes in necrotizing fasciitis are generally more severe and are found in deeper layers, with fluid tracking along the deep fascia.[37]

Peripheral vein septic thrombophlebitis may present similarly to a cutaneous abscess and cellulitis. The sonographic findings of peripheral vein septic thrombophlebitis include a noncompressible vein with an anechoic or echogenic thrombus within the lumen, vessel wall thickening, and lack of color Doppler flow[37] (**Fig. 27**).

SOFT-TISSUE FOREIGN BODIES
Overview

Soft-tissue foreign bodies (STFBs) are usually caused by puncture or impalement injuries and are frequently evaluated by primary care physicians in the clinical setting. STFBs may consist of variable compositions, including metal, wood, plastic, glass, cement, or stone. Traditionally, these materials are classified into 2 categories—radiopaque or radiolucent—based on whether they can be seen on x-ray. Wood, thorn, plastic, nail slivers, rubber, and glass may be radiolucent and missed with x-ray.[43] Fortunately, ultrasound is reliable for detecting these radiolucent STFBs.[44]

The sonographic findings of STFBs are variable depending on composition and location. Size, shape, injury mechanism, retained duration, prior exploration, local

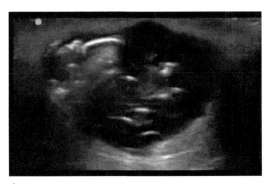

Fig. 26. Soft tissue abscess.

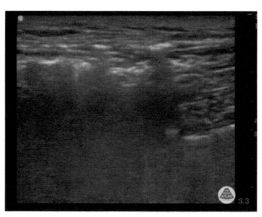

Fig. 27. Gas in soft tissue. Hyperechoic gas (screen left) obscures the typical architecture of soft tissues (screen right). There is a small amount of edema in the superficial soft tissues. (*From* thepocusatlas.com; with permission.)

inflammatory changes, and air trapping may all impact STFB appearance on ultrasound (**Box 2**).

Scanning for STFBs

Foreign bodies can be small and difficult to detect. A careful and methodological evaluation is essential. Scanning from multiple angles and scanning the contralateral side for comparison are useful strategies. At times, cine-loop analysis, in which a sequence of digital frames of images are acquired and viewed in slow motion can assist in detecting small foreign bodies. The use of power Doppler imaging may aid in detection by increasing the conspicuity of both the hypoechoic halo and the foreign body itself.[46] When an FB is detected, it is advised to identify its longitudinal axis by rotating the probe to variable degrees and to mark the skin to assist future scans or removal.

Ultrasound-Guided STFB Removal

Ultrasound-guided foreign body removal in an experienced hand has a high success rate close to 90% based on a large case series.[47] The key to success is using a systomic approach and to approach foreign bodies methodically.

Before attempting FB removal, scan the affected area in at least 2 orientations to make sure that there are not multiple FBs present. Once an FB is detected, adjust the probe to obtain its longitudinal axis view and note its depth in relation to the

---

Box 2
Common findings in STFB

1. All STFBs are echogenic.

2. Shadowing and reverberation artifacts are commonly seen.

3. A hypoechoic halo may surround the foreign body if a significant infectious/inflammatory process has ensued.

4. Surrounding soft tissue or structural changes as well as bleeding, infection, or air trapping can be observed[45] (**Fig. 28**).

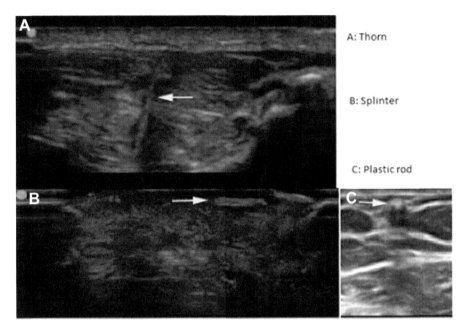

A: Thorn

B: Splinter

C: Plastic rod

Fig. 28. Foreign body on ultrasound.

skin.[48] Mark the location, longitudinal orientation, and the most superficial end of the FB. If there is an open wound, irrigate it with sterile saline and scan the FB again to make sure no migration occurred. Prep the targeted area with a proper skin cleanser. For superficial FBs, direct ultrasound guidance may not be needed and a simple incision at the superficial end of the FB as determined by ultrasound might be enough for extraction.[47] However, for deeper FBs, ultrasound guidance proves to be helpful. Under sterile fashion, with a sterile ultrasound probe cover, sterile gel, and possible sterile gel standoff pad, a HFL probe is used to obtain a longitudinal axis view of the FB. Under real-time imaging in an in-plane mode, consider using a finder needle[49,50] to locate the foreign body at the most superficial end. If a finder needle is used, try to insert it as close to the FB as possible. Then, use an 11 sized scalpel blade to make an incision that is large enough to allow crocodile forceps or mosquito-type forceps to enter and operate. Using the blunt dissection technique under direct guidance, advance the forceps to the superficial end of the FB.[51] Once the location is reached, open the forceps to grasp the FB under ultrasound guidance. Once the FB is secured on the forceps, retract the instrument to remove the FB. Irrigate the wound with sterile saline. Close the incision if the wound is deemed to be clean. Otherwise, consider leaving it open to heal by second intention. Dress the wound properly and update the patient's tetanus status if needed. Consider antibiotics prophylaxis for chronic or dirty wounds.

CLINICS CARE POINTS

US-guided MSK injection:
- When performing ultrasound-guided injection, arrange yourself, the patient, and the ultrasound machine in a straight line, in that order, so that you can visualize the injection site and the ultrasound image without turning your head.

Cardiac:

- When performing cardiac POCUS, it may be necessary to have the patient in the left lateral decubitus position to improve visualization, by bringing the heart closer to the chest wall, especially for patients with large body habitus and/or chronic obstructive pulmonary disease.

DVT:
- For patients with low pretest probability, DVT can be ruled out with 2-point compression ultrasound without measuring a D-dimer.

AAA:
- When screening for AAA using POCUS, be sure to visualize the proximal, mid, and distal abdominal aorta in both transverse and longitudinal orientations, to catch both saccular and fusiform aneurysms.

Soft-tissue:
- Patients with cellulitis will have characteristic cobblestoning on ultrasound, but this finding is not specific for cellulitis and can be seen in other conditions associated with edema.

DISCLOSURE

The authors have nothing to disclose.

SUPPLEMENTARY DATA

Supplementary data related to this article can be found online at 10.1016/j.pop.2021. 10.011.

REFERENCES

1. Al Deeb M, Barbic S, Featherstone R, et al. Point-of-care ultrasonography for the diagnosis of acute cardiogenic pulmonary edema in patients presenting with acute dyspnea: a systematic review and meta-analysis. Acad Emerg Med 2014;21(8):843–52.
2. Melniker LA, Leibner E, McKenney MG, et al. Randomized controlled clinical trial of point-of-care, limited ultrasonography for trauma in the emergency department: the first sonography outcomes assessment program trial. Ann Emerg Med 2006;48(3):227–35.
3. Parker L, Nazarian LN, Carrino JA, et al. Musculoskeletal imaging: medicare use, costs, and potential for cost substitution. J Am Coll Radiol 2008;5(3):182–8.
4. Smith-Bindman R, Aubin C, Bailitz J, et al. Ultrasonography versus computed tomography for suspected nephrolithiasis. N Engl J Med 2014;371(12):1100–10.
5. Glazier RH, Dalby DM, Badley EM, et al. Determinants of physician confidence in the primary care management of musculoskeletal disorders. J Rheumatol 1996; 23(2):351–6.
6. De Zordo T, Mur E, Bellmann-Weiler R, et al. US guided injections in arthritis. Eur J Radiol 2009;71(2):197–203.
7. Lawson A, Kelsberg G, Safranek S. Clinical inquiry. Does ultrasound guidance improve outcomes for steroid joint injections? Yes, at least in the short term. J Fam Pract 2013;62(12). 763a-763c.
8. Pourcho AM, Colio SW, Hall MM. Ultrasound-Guided Interventional Procedures About the Shoulder: Anatomy, Indications, and Techniques. Phys Med Rehabil Clin N Am 2016;27(3):555–72.
9. Lee JY, Park Y, Park KD, et al. Effectiveness of ultrasound-guided carpal tunnel injection using in-plane ulnar approach: a prospective, randomized, single-blinded study. Medicine (Baltimore) 2014;93(29):e350.

10. Colio SW, Smith J, Pourcho AM. Ultrasound-Guided Interventional Procedures of the Wrist and Hand: Anatomy, Indications, and Techniques. Phys Med Rehabil Clin N Am 2016;27(3):589–605.
11. Rowbotham EL, Grainger AJ. Ultrasound-guided intervention around the hip joint. AJR Am J Roentgenol 2011;197(1):W122–7.
12. Murray T, Roberts D, Rattan B, et al. Dynamic ultrasound-guided trochanteric bursal injection. Skeletal Radiol 2020;49(7):1155–8.
13. Lueders DR, Smith J, Sellon JL. Ultrasound-Guided Knee Procedures. Phys Med Rehabil Clin N Am 2016;27(3):631–48.
14. Sahler CS, Spinner DA, Kirschner JS. Ultrasound-guided first metatarsophalangeal joint injections: description of an in-plane, gel standoff technique in a cadaveric study. Foot Ankle Spec 2013;6(4):303–6.
15. Feigenbaum H. Evolution of echocardiography. Circulation 1996;93(7):1321–7.
16. Croft LB, Duvall WL, Goldman ME. A pilot study of the clinical impact of hand-carried cardiac ultrasound in the medical clinic. Echocardiography 2006;23(6):439–46.
17. Lucas BP, Candotti C, Margeta B, et al. Diagnostic accuracy of hospitalist-performed hand-carried ultrasound echocardiography after a brief training program. J Hosp Med 2009;4(6):340–9.
18. Melamed R, Sprenkle MD, Ulstad VK, et al. Assessment of left ventricular function by intensivists using hand-held echocardiography. Chest 2009;135(6):1416–20.
19. Vignon P, Dugard A, Abraham J, et al. Focused training for goal-oriented hand-held echocardiography performed by noncardiologist residents in the intensive care unit. Intensive Care Med 2007;33(10):1795–9.
20. Kimura BJ. Point-of-care cardiac ultrasound techniques in the physical examination: better at the bedside. Heart 2017;103(13):987–94.
21. Kimura BJ, Shaw DJ, Amundson SA, et al. Cardiac Limited Ultrasound Examination Techniques to Augment the Bedside Cardiac Physical Examination. J Ultrasound Med 2015;34(9):1683–90.
22. Bouzas-Mosquera A, Broullón FJ, Álvarez-García N, et al. Left atrial size and risk for all-cause mortality and ischemic stroke. CMAJ 2011;183(10):E657–64.
23. Kimura BJ, Kedar E, Weiss DE, et al. A bedside ultrasound sign of cardiac disease: the left atrium-to-aorta diastolic diameter ratio. Am J Emerg Med 2010; 28(2):203–7.
24. Burnside PR, Brown MD, Kline JA. Systematic review of emergency physician-performed ultrasonography for lower-extremity deep vein thrombosis. Acad Emerg Med 2008;15(6):493–8.
25. Lee JH, Lee SH, Yun SJ. Comparison of 2-point and 3-point point-of-care ultrasound techniques for deep vein thrombosis at the emergency department: A meta-analysis. Medicine (Baltimore) 2019;98(22):e15791.
26. Cogo A, Lensing AW, Koopman MM, et al. Compression ultrasonography for diagnostic management of patients with clinically suspected deep vein thrombosis: prospective cohort study. BMJ 1998;316(7124):17–20.
27. Ageno W, Camporese G, Riva N, et al. Analysis of an algorithm incorporating limited and whole-leg assessment of the deep venous system in symptomatic outpatients with suspected deep-vein thrombosis (PALLADIO): a prospective, multicentre, cohort study. Lancet Haematol 2015;2(11):e474–80.
28. Bornemann P, Jayasekera N, Bergman K, et al. Point-of-care ultrasound: Coming soon to primary care? J Fam Pract 2018;67(2):70–80.
29. Guirguis-Blake JM, Beil TL, Senger CA, et al. Primary Care Screening for Abdominal Aortic Aneurysm: Updated Evidence Report and Systematic Review for the US Preventive Services Task Force. JAMA 2019;322(22):2219–38.

30. O'Donnell TFX, Landon BE, Schermerhorn ML. AAA Screening Should Be Expanded. Circulation 2019;140(11):889–90.

31. Rubano E, Mehta N, Caputo W, et al. Systematic review: emergency department bedside ultrasonography for diagnosing suspected abdominal aortic aneurysm. Acad Emerg Med 2013;20(2):128–38.

32. Martindale JL, Wakai A, Collins SP, et al. Diagnosing Acute Heart Failure in the Emergency Department: A Systematic Review and Meta-analysis. Acad Emerg Med 2016;23(3):223–42.

33. Xia Y, Ying Y, Wang S, et al. Effectiveness of lung ultrasonography for diagnosis of pneumonia in adults: a systematic review and meta-analysis. J Thorac Dis 2016; 8(10):2822–31.

34. Yousefifard M, Baikpour M, Ghelichkhani P, et al. Screening Performance Characteristic of Ultrasonography and Radiography in Detection of Pleural Effusion; a Meta-Analysis. Emerg (Tehran) 2016;4(1):1–10.

35. Alsaawi A, Alrajhi K, Alshehri A, et al. Ultrasonography for the diagnosis of patients with clinically suspected skin and soft tissue infections: a systematic review of the literature. Eur J Emerg Med 2017;24(3):162–9.

36. Tayal VS, Hasan N, Norton HJ, et al. The effect of soft-tissue ultrasound on the management of cellulitis in the emergency department. Acad Emerg Med 2006;13(4):384–8.

37. Adhikari S, Blaivas M. Sonography first for subcutaneous abscess and cellulitis evaluation. J Ultrasound Med 2012;31(10):1509–12.

38. Comer AB. Point-of-Care Ultrasound for Skin and Soft Tissue Infections. Adv Emerg Nurs J 2018;40(4):296–303.

39. Gottlieb M, Avila J, Chottiner M, et al. Point-of-Care Ultrasonography for the Diagnosis of Skin and Soft Tissue Abscesses: A Systematic Review and Meta-analysis. Ann Emerg Med 2020;76(1):67–77.

40. Lam SHF, Sivitz A, Alade K, et al. Comparison of Ultrasound Guidance vs. Clinical Assessment Alone for Management of Pediatric Skin and Soft Tissue Infections. J Emerg Med 2018;55(5):693–701.

41. Gaspari RJ, Blehar D, Polan D, et al. The Massachusetts abscess rule: a clinical decision rule using ultrasound to identify methicillin-resistant Staphylococcus aureus in skin abscesses. Acad Emerg Med 2014;21(5):558–67.

42. Butcher CH, Dooley RW, Levitov AB. Detection of subcutaneous and intramuscular air with sonography: a sensitive and specific modality. J Ultrasound Med 2011;30(6):791–5.

43. Tantray MD, Rather A, Manaan Q, et al. Role of ultrasound in detection of radiolucent foreign bodies in extremities. Strateg Trauma Limb Reconstr 2018;13(2):81–5.

44. Ginsburg MJ, Ellis GL, Flom LL. Detection of soft-tissue foreign bodies by plain radiography, xerography, computed tomography, and ultrasonography. Ann Emerg Med 1990;19(6):701–3.

45. Boyse TD, Fessell DP, Jacobson JA, et al. US of soft-tissue foreign bodies and associated complications with surgical correlation. Radiographics 2001;21(5):1251–6.

46. Davae KC, Sofka CM, DiCarlo E, et al. Value of power Doppler imaging and the hypoechoic halo in the sonographic detection of foreign bodies: correlation with histopathologic findings. J Ultrasound Med 2003;22(12):1309–13.

47. Bradley M. Image-guided soft-tissue foreign body extraction - success and pitfalls. Clin Radiol 2012;67(6):531–4.

48. Lulla A, Whitman T, Amii R, et al. Role of Ultrasound in the Identification of Longitudinal Axis in Soft-Tissue Foreign Body Extraction. West J Emerg Med 2016;17(6):819–21.

49. Nwawka OK, Kabutey NK, Locke CM, et al. Ultrasound-guided needle localization to aid foreign body removal in pediatric patients. J Foot Ankle Surg 2014;53(1):67–70.
50. Porter MD, Schriver JP. Ultrasound-guided Kopans' needle location and removal of a retained foreign body. Surg Endosc 2000;14(5):500.
51. Paziana K, Fields JM, Rotte M, et al. Soft tissue foreign body removal technique using portable ultrasonography. Wilderness Environ Med 2012;23(4):343–8.

9780323809191